W0018475

The Lost Generation of COVID-19

The COVID-19 pandemic has wrought unparalleled disruption, altering the landscape of health and well-being for a generation. *The Lost Generation of COVID-19* unveils the ways in which the crisis has deepened existing health disparities, casting a long shadow over young people's futures.

Set against the backdrop of austerity-induced cuts to UK public services, this book explores the social determinants of health, revealing how systemic neglect has been exacerbated by the pandemic's relentless pressure. The analysis extends beyond individual hardships, illuminating the broader societal ramifications such as economic stagnation and social fragmentation. Yet, amidst the bleak landscape, the book offers a visionary perspective on the potential for transformative change. It posits that the pandemic serves as a catalyst for radical societal reform, advocating for a new economic paradigm anchored in equity and fairness. By addressing the root causes of health inequalities through innovative policy interventions and structural reforms, the author envisions a resilient and just society emerging from the shadows of the pandemic.

Insightful and far-reaching, this book is an indispensable resource for students and scholars in the health sciences and political science, as well as for policymakers dedicated to these important issues.

Jatinder Hayre is an established public health academic and medical doctor recognised for his innovative research on health inequalities and social determinants of health. He has authored numerous influential and authoritative publications and led key studies that have informed national health policy in the UK. A respected grassroots campaigner, Dr Hayre seamlessly integrates academia, clinical practice, and campaigns for social good: driving transformative initiatives towards a more equitable and just society.

The Lost Generation of COVID-19

A Critical Analysis of Health and Social Inequality in Post-Pandemic Britain

Jatinder Hayre

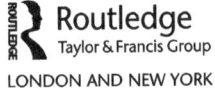

Routledge
Taylor & Francis Group

LONDON AND NEW YORK

First published 2025
by Routledge
4 Park Square, Milton Park, Abingdon, Oxon OX14 4RN

and by Routledge
605 Third Avenue, New York, NY 10158

Routledge is an imprint of the Taylor & Francis Group, an informa business

© 2025 Jatinder Hayre

The right of Jatinder Hayre to be identified as author of this work has been asserted in accordance with sections 77 and 78 of the Copyright, Designs and Patents Act 1988.

All rights reserved. No part of this book may be reprinted or reproduced or utilised in any form or by any electronic, mechanical, or other means, now known or hereafter invented, including photocopying and recording, or in any information storage or retrieval system, without permission in writing from the publishers.

Trademark notice: Product or corporate names may be trademarks or registered trademarks, and are used only for identification and explanation without intent to infringe.

British Library Cataloguing-in-Publication Data
A catalogue record for this book is available from the British Library

ISBN: 978-1-032-32045-8 (hbk)
ISBN: 978-1-041-06287-5 (pbk)
ISBN: 978-1-003-31252-9 (ebk)

DOI: 10.4324/9781003312529

Typeset in Times New Roman
by Apex CoVantage LLC

Contents

About the Author

Dr Jatinder Hayre's roots trace back to the industrious Black Country, where he was raised by hardworking parents: his mother, a dedicated cleaner, and his father, a scrap metalworker. Growing up in this close-knit, working-class community instilled in Dr Hayre a deep appreciation for resilience, solidarity, and the importance of fighting for social justice.

Inspired by his upbringing, Jatinder pursued a career in medicine, earning national recognition as an award-winning medical doctor. His clinical practice, grounded in compassion and a commitment to equity, naturally extended into his research endeavours. As a leading researcher in health and social inequalities, Jatinder has made significant contributions to understanding and addressing the systemic factors that perpetuate disparities in health outcomes.

One of his notable achievements includes leading the Independent SAGE report on "COVID-19 and Health Inequality", which played a crucial role in influencing government policy to reverse cuts to Universal Credit during the pandemic. This work exemplifies his ability to bridge clinical insights with impactful policy advocacy, ensuring that vulnerable populations receive the support they need.

Beyond his professional and academic pursuits, Jatinder is a dedicated campaigner and trade unionist. Serving as the national spokesperson for Keep Our NHS Public, he tirelessly advocates for health equity and justice. His long-standing involvement as Vice Director of the Socialist Health Association and work within The Fabian Society think tank has been instrumental in shaping progressive health policies and driving meaningful campaigns.

In this book, Dr Hayre draws on his extensive experience to explore the enduring impacts of the pandemic on youth and societal health disparities. His thoughtful analysis not only highlights the challenges but also envisions pathways towards a more equitable and resilient society.

Rooted in his working-class background and driven by a lifelong desire to make a material difference, Dr Jatinder Hayre's work continues to examine the pressing issues of health inequality, inspiring both his peers and the next generation to strive for a fairer and healthier future for all.

Introduction

Britain's protracted struggle with COVID-19 has fundamentally reshaped its social, economic, and health landscape. The pandemic has often been hailed as a "great leveller", but closer scrutiny reveals the deep cracks in a society long marked by entrenched inequities. From the stories of frontline workers grappling with inadequate resources to the disadvantaged communities left without robust social protection, the virus latched onto—and sometimes worsened—long-standing vulnerabilities. At the heart of these struggles lies the "Lost Generation": individuals who bore the brunt of pandemic lockdowns, economic downturns, and systemic inequalities. The chapters that follow in this book underscore the multiple dimensions of Britain's post-pandemic reality, focusing on disparities that were neither created nor resolved by COVID-19 but thrust into sharper relief by the crisis. This introduction aims to provide a critical overview of the themes explored, painting a picture of how and why certain groups have been left behind, and what that signifies for the future of a country still reeling from the reverberations of an unprecedented global event.

From the start, the British government's public health response faced immense pressure to balance economic imperatives with the lives and livelihoods of its citizens. Yet even the earliest debates about when to institute or relax lockdowns were often informed by competing priorities: rescuing a flailing economy or protecting the NHS from being overwhelmed. This tension laid bare the stark social inequalities that already divided the country. Individuals with insecure work contracts found themselves forced to choose between their personal health and their limited financial safety nets, a dilemma that rarely plagued those with salaried, stable employment. In regions that were already economically disadvantaged, the disruptive force of COVID-19 was amplified tenfold, leaving communities ill-equipped to cope with or recover from successive waves of infection. While the chapters on policy response dig deeper into government decision-making, it is evident that the interplay of austerity measures, political discourse, and public trust in state institutions significantly contributed to how the pandemic unfolded for distinct groups.

DOI: 10.4324/9781003312529-1

The first substantive chapters in this volume highlight how racial and ethnic minorities were disproportionately affected, in terms of both health outcomes and broader socioeconomic impact. Pre-existing health inequalities—rooted in structural discrimination, reduced access to high-quality healthcare, and limited health-seeking behaviours—set the stage for elevated mortality rates among Black, Asian, and other minority ethnic communities. Underlying factors ranged from overcrowded living conditions to widespread job insecurity, with many individuals in these communities employed in front-facing roles that left them at higher risk of viral exposure. Despite widespread acknowledgement of these issues by health agencies and community groups, interventions have often been piecemeal or reactionary, struggling to keep pace with the continuous onslaught of rising infection rates and evolving variants. The chapters delve into how cultural mistrust of state institutions, coupled with inadequate health communication campaigns, eroded adherence to official guidelines. They argue that without deliberate, inclusive strategies, the legacy of COVID-19 will remain etched in statistics that show tragically higher fatality rates for marginalised populations.

Equally pressing is the plight of children and young people who found their formative years interrupted by prolonged school closures, sporadic virtual learning, and stunted social development. A generation that should have been preoccupied with forging social bonds, mastering new skills, and dreaming of future careers faced a barrage of uncertainty, isolation, and anxiety. The chapters on education and youth inequality illustrate how the loss of face-to-face instruction widened attainment gaps, with disadvantaged students falling further behind their more privileged peers. While digital learning tools served as a stopgap measure, they could not replicate the breadth of academic, social, and emotional support systems provided within physical schools. Lacking adequate technology or study space at home, many pupils in lower-income households were simply unable to keep pace. Children from families already grappling with food insecurity faced deepening hardships as free school meals and other support mechanisms were disrupted, sowing the seeds for chronic educational deficits and long-term socioeconomic consequences. These chapters collectively illustrate that the label "Lost Generation" is no hyperbole when it comes to Britain's youth. The book posits that the intergenerational effects of these lost opportunities will reverberate far beyond the immediate aftermath of the pandemic.

Economic fragilities constitute another crucial lens through which to view the COVID-19 crisis. Wage freezes, furlough schemes, and unprecedented job losses all contributed to a shifting and increasingly precarious employment landscape. The pandemic, for many, exposed just how few had genuine financial resilience. Renters struggled under the threat of eviction, freelance and gig-economy workers found themselves abruptly left with no income, and entire sectors such as hospitality and tourism faced near collapse. The macroeconomic chapters in this book detail the fault lines in Britain's labour market, suggesting that the abrupt shock of the pandemic served as a stress test for a system already stretched to its limits by automation, global competition, and years of austerity. For the so-called "Lost Generation", these changes may set the trajectory of an entire lifetime of diminished earning potential and precarious job prospects, not to mention the emotional toll of long-term unemployment or underemployment. In painting this stark picture, the authors challenge readers to consider whether the country's current economic frameworks can be reimagined in ways that are equitable and resilient in the face of new crises yet to come.

A salient theme throughout the chapters is the ripple effect of mental health challenges. By the time COVID-19 reached Britain's shores, services for mental health were already under strain, with long waiting lists, shortages of qualified professionals, and funding that trailed far behind demand. The pandemic exacerbated this shortfall on multiple fronts. Healthcare workers reported experiencing acute burnout, as they battled surges of patients alongside the anxiety of exposing their own families to the virus. Children, isolated from their peer groups and facing persistent uncertainty around examinations and future prospects, reported heightened rates of stress, depression, and suicidal ideation. Young adults, who might ordinarily have been forging connections at university or entering the workforce, found themselves stuck at home, sometimes contending with familial conflicts and an uncertain economy. Across these pages, one finds compelling discussions on how the mental health crisis not only emerged from COVID-19 but also mirrored and magnified the structural inequities that originally hampered service provision. The chapters argue that an adequate policy response must prioritise mental health not as an afterthought but as a cornerstone of pandemic recovery. Only then might Britain begin to alleviate the profound suffering of individuals already burdened by other forms of inequality.

British society's most vulnerable populations—homeless individuals, asylum seekers, those with disabilities, and the elderly—featured heavily in the grim statistics that poured in daily. Their stories occupy an important place in this book, illustrating not only the immediate crisis they faced but also how institutional frameworks often failed to offer meaningful protection. Care homes, for instance, became focal points of tragedy, with systemic flaws in safety protocols leading to disproportionate mortality among older adults. Similarly, those who were already homeless found their precarious existence rendered even more perilous by public health directives they had little means to follow. The chapters on marginalised groups confront readers with uncomfortable truths: a pandemic does not bestow universal vulnerability; it exacerbates the vulnerabilities that already exist. They also challenge any notion that such adversities could be resolved by charitable acts alone. Rather, the authors argue for systemic reforms, grounded in an equitable understanding of social and health policy, to ensure that vulnerable populations are not consigned to the fringes of society as the country rebuilds.

Underpinning all these discussions is a persistent thread: the notion of collective responsibility versus individual autonomy. Britain's discourse on masks, vaccines, and lockdowns often revolved around the tension between personal freedoms and the welfare of the wider community. These debates were shaped by political narratives that framed state intervention as either paternalistic overreach or a necessary measure to prevent mass casualties. The chapters exploring public attitudes and media representations reveal how societal fault lines—race, class, and geography—were exploited by competing ideologies. The polarisation of public sentiment made it increasingly difficult to adopt interventions that were both effective and equitable. Vaccine hesitancy, a focus of one of the chapters, emerged at the intersection of mistrust in political institutions, fear of side effects, and the widespread dissemination of misinformation. Throughout these debates, certain demographic groups were subtly vilified for allegedly hindering the return to "normalcy". By examining these tensions, the book underscores the complexity of orchestrating a unified response in a fragmented society, and how that fragmentation persists in post-pandemic Britain.

By illuminating these multiple intersecting crises—health, education, economic precarity, mental health, and social cohesion—the book asks whether Britain is willing to confront the lessons of COVID-19 or simply move on. The official narrative promoting recovery often defaults to celebratory language about "resilience" and "bounce-back". This runs the risk of glossing over the enduring inequalities that the pandemic exposed. The final chapters propose a roadmap for rethinking Britain's social contract, arguing that if we fail to address the structural underpinnings of inequality, future crises will merely entrench them further. Policy recommendations span a spectrum of possibilities, from reforming the welfare system to providing sustainable funding for mental health services, from recalibrating employment policies to ensuring that public health communication is culturally attuned and linguistically accessible. The question is not merely how to fix what is broken but how to imagine a society in which no group is systematically left behind.

Thus, the term "Lost Generation" resonates not only with the immediate experiences of those who have struggled through the pandemic but also with the looming prospect of prolonged disadvantage. The focus in these pages is on Britain, but the issues raised—the fragility of labour markets, racial and class disparities, the flaws in public health infrastructure, and the mental health toll of prolonged collective trauma—reflect broader global patterns. Yet Britain's unique historical, socio-political, and institutional context lends its own character to this crisis and its aftermath. Through detailed case studies, policy analyses, and personal accounts, the chapters that follow construct a comprehensive picture of the pandemic's multilayered impact. They also prompt readers to ask: How will future generations judge the political choices and societal norms that shaped Britain's pandemic response? Who will be remembered as the most vulnerable, and did we do enough to protect them?

Were communities equipped to stand together, or did we fracture further along existing fault lines?

In presenting this introduction, the aim is not merely to recount the enormous toll of COVID-19 in Britain but to situate these events within a longer arc of social inequality and political decisions that have defined the country's modern history. The "Lost Generation", in this context, becomes a symbol of unfulfilled promises, of delayed or derailed aspirations, and of a society more aware than ever of its deep divisions. Over the subsequent chapters, the book delves into each dimension of inequality, weaving together data-driven analyses and personal narratives to illustrate how COVID-19 transformed individual lives and collective identities. It invites readers to consider the lessons that might be gleaned—and how those lessons can be acted upon as Britain forges its post-pandemic path. In short, *The Lost Generation of COVID-19: A Critical Analysis of Health and Social Inequality in Post-Pandemic* Britain tells a story of rupture and revelation, urging us to acknowledge the profound imbalances that threaten not just the health of individuals but the future of an entire nation.

1 Education

Introduction

Education stands at the heart of human progress, both as a process and as a product. The process of education engages the individual in acquiring, questioning, and applying knowledge—a developmental journey that unfolds across childhood and adolescence. The product of education, in turn, signifies the accumulation of cognitive skills, social competencies, and personal dispositions that shape life trajectories, adult well-being, and social identity. This dual nature of education is acutely relevant to public health: research consistently demonstrates that educational engagement and attainment influence not only cognitive development and future socioeconomic standing but also health outcomes ranging from chronic disease prevalence to overall life expectancy (1–5).

Nevertheless, the transformative power of education is neither uniformly distributed nor automatically guaranteed. Societies stratified by income, geography, and political history frequently exhibit vast disparities in educational access and quality—disparities that further translate into long-term health and social inequities. In the UK, the period of austerity from 2010 to 2019 substantially undermined public investment in schooling, particularly in the most deprived areas. This decade of systemic underfunding coincided with and exacerbated long-standing educational divides. Children from disadvantaged backgrounds felt the impact from their earliest years of life: nursery closures and depleted early childhood services left them ill-prepared for formal schooling, compounding inequities that grew with each stage of education.

When COVID-19 arrived in early 2020, these existing fissures became chasms. School closures, remote learning, and the "digital divide" locked the poorest families out of equitable educational opportunities, pushing a fractured system to the brink. Disadvantaged children, especially those without reliable devices or dedicated study space, fell irretrievably behind their better-resourced peers. The consequences of such educational losses are not merely academic: they affect children's mental health, physical well-being, and life chances in ways that will echo for decades. This chapter presents

DOI: 10.4324/9781003312529-2

a critical, in-depth analysis of how these patterns of educational inequality emerged, how they worsened under austerity, and how the pandemic laid bare the existing fractures—thereby endangering the health and futures of Britain's youth.

1.1 Conceptual Foundations: Education as a Social Determinant of Health

1.1.1 Education: Process and Product

Education has traditionally been understood as a linear progression of formal learning—from early childhood programmes through primary and secondary schooling, culminating in higher or further education. Yet such a narrow perspective risks obscuring the broader significance of education as both a process and a product (1). The educational process fosters critical thinking, social skills, self-efficacy, and resilience—traits that weave into every dimension of daily life. The product of education, meanwhile, manifests in the qualifications, credentials, and competencies that define employability, earning potential, and social capital.

In public health research, these distinctions are crucial. Studies underscore that individuals with greater educational attainment tend to have better control of blood pressure, lower smoking rates, and improved self-rated health (2,3). They also have lower rates of chronic conditions like diabetes and cardiovascular disease (2). Viewed in this light, education is both a buffer against immediate health risks—through enhanced health literacy and reduced engagement in unhealthy behaviours—and a pathway to higher-income employment, stronger social networks, and improved access to healthcare resources (4,5).

1.1.2 The Triple Benefit: Physical, Mental, and Social Well-Being

The 1978 Alma-Ata Declaration redefined health as "a state of complete physical, mental and social well-being". By that measure, education contributes to all three domains, reinforcing the holistic nature of wellness. Physically, higher educational attainment correlates with better management of risk factors for chronic disease. Mentally, the cognitive and emotional competencies cultivated in school support resilience, self-regulation, and stress management. Socially, educational institutions facilitate peer connection, social belonging, and the accumulation of cultural capital that can protect against isolation and marginalisation.

Recent findings have shown that raising the minimum school-leaving age can lead to measurable improvements in health outcomes, including mental health, functional independence in older age, and self-reported quality of life (5). These benefits underscore the premise that formal education, especially when extended or made more inclusive, can be a prophylactic measure against future morbidity and mortality.

1.1.3   Education and Intergenerational Social Mobility

Beyond these immediate effects on individual health, education functions as a lever for intergenerational social mobility. Qualifications open doors to higher-paying careers, creating a ripple effect that benefits entire families. This intergenerational dividend becomes particularly pronounced in communities that experience entrenched poverty. When children acquire robust educational outcomes, they break cycles of deprivation—thereby enhancing opportunities for their own offspring to access better resources, live in healthier neighbourhoods, and perpetuate upward trajectories.

However, these potent advantages hinge on equitable access to quality education. Where schooling is underfunded or socioeconomically stratified, the very children who could most benefit from an educational safety net are often those who remain excluded or poorly served. Historically, Britain's policy framework, dating back to the landmark Beveridge Report of 1942, aimed to tackle the "giants" of social harm, including ignorance. Nevertheless, the subsequent decades have exposed a disturbing persistence—and even entrenchment—of educational inequity.

1.2   The Legacy of the Beveridge Report: Ignorance as a Societal Ill

1.2.1   Beveridge's Vision and Contemporary Realities

In 1942, Sir William Beveridge identified five "Giant Evils": Want, Disease, Ignorance, Squalor, and Idleness. By classifying "ignorance" as a societal ill, the Beveridge Report acknowledged that a lack of education leads to poor life outcomes—not merely for individuals but for the collective well-being of society. From a contemporary vantage point, the challenge remains startlingly similar: subpar education constrains opportunity, entrenches inequality, and erodes the foundations of a healthy populace.

Although the post-war establishment of free, compulsory education signalled a monumental step forward, the decades that followed revealed enduring deficits. Educational policy improvements tended to lag behind shifting demographic realities, regional disparities, and waves of economic pressure. Today, the "giant of Ignorance" persists in the form of stark attainment gaps, illiteracy pockets, and long waiting lists for special educational needs assessments—a testament to an education system that continues to fail many of the most vulnerable children.

1.2.2 The Rise (and Fall) of Post-War Social Optimism

Following World War II, Britain embarked on a robust campaign of social reform. Alongside the founding of the National Health Service, improvements in education were considered crucial to forging a healthier, more equitable society. For much of the 20th century, expansions in comprehensive schooling, an increase in higher education enrolment, and greater resource allocation to deprived areas represented attempts to realise Beveridge's vision.

However, fluctuations in political will and economic fortunes meant these efforts were neither linear nor uniform. Over time, pressures to reduce public spending—and a growing emphasis on "localism" and market-based education—contributed to uneven outcomes. By the dawn of the 21st century, it became evident that, while universal schooling had lifted educational levels across the nation, major disparities in funding, teaching quality, and pupil support endured.

1.2.3 The Contemporary Challenge of Ignorance

Today's "giant of Ignorance" diverges from Beveridge's 1940s-era concerns in certain respects—digital literacy, technological disruptions, and global competition intensify the stakes—but the underlying problem remains. Children born into under-resourced neighbourhoods, with parents experiencing unemployment or unstable incomes, typically face substantial barriers to success. For them, education can be an exit route from generational poverty, but only if accompanied by holistic investments in early childhood, learning infrastructure, and ongoing welfare support. Lacking these, the link between deprivation and poor health becomes further entrenched, propagating inequality across generations.

1.3 Austerity Britain (2010–2019): Eroding the Foundations

1.3.1 Austerity's Emergence and Policy Framework

In the wake of the 2008 global financial crisis, successive UK governments implemented austerity measures to reduce public sector deficits. These policies entailed significant cuts in public expenditure, encompassing welfare budgets, local authority grants, and sectoral funding for education. Officials justified austerity on the grounds of fiscal discipline; however, critics argued that such measures effectively weakened the societal safety net, with vulnerable populations shouldering a disproportionate burden.

For education, the ramifications were stark. While schools in affluent areas experienced moderate or, in some cases, marginal funding reductions, those in the most deprived localities faced per-pupil cuts nearing 9% (6). The effect on day-to-day school life was immediate and visible: larger class sizes, fewer teaching assistants, reduced extracurricular offerings, and dwindling resources for special educational needs.

1.3.2   The Erosion of the Pupil Premium

Instituted to tackle disadvantage and narrow the attainment gap, the Pupil Premium provided schools with additional funds for students eligible for free school meals. Initially lauded as a beacon of progressive policy, the Pupil Premium soon lost its real-term value under austerity, declining by around 8% between 2014 and 2018 (7). As inflation and student enrolments rose, the nominal funding remained the same—forcing schools to stretch resources even further.

This diminution severely undermined the Premium's intended purpose. Extra support such as tutoring, nutritional programmes, or counselling, which could have broken cycles of underachievement, became unsustainable in many cases. Crucially, this shortfall was felt most acutely by the very children who relied on these services, entrenching disadvantage even before the pandemic hit.

1.3.3   The Widening Attainment Gap

By 2019, children from economically marginalised backgrounds were, on average, 18.1 months behind their more affluent peers upon completion of their General Certificate of Secondary Education (GCSE) exams—an alarming gap that begins in primary school, where it already stands at roughly 9.3 months (8). This evidence testifies that educational inequality is not a sudden phenomenon emerging in adolescence; rather, it is seeded in the earliest years of life.

Such disparities inevitably carry profound implications for both individual and societal health. Pupils exiting secondary school with lower qualifications face limited pathways to vocational training or higher education, thus perpetuating cycles of low-paid or precarious employment. As research attests, these precarious socioeconomic prospects correlate strongly with poorer health outcomes, from reduced self-rated health to an elevated risk of chronic disease (2,4).

1.3.4   Slashing Early Childhood Services

Austerity measures affected more than primary and secondary schooling: they also targeted early years support. Local authorities cut an average of £532 per child from early childhood education budgets between 2010 and

2018 (8). This funding had often underpinned children's centres, nursery provision, and parenting programmes. Eliminating or diminishing these services not only undermined child development but also curtailed crucial support for families grappling with unemployment, housing insecurity, or mental health challenges.

The result was a cohort of children entering the formal education system with developmental gaps in language, emotional regulation, and social skills—gaps that can be extremely difficult to close in later years. For parents, especially single parents or those with multiple jobs, the loss of subsidised childcare made it harder to maintain stable employment. These family-level stresses cascade into children's daily lives, further complicating their ability to engage and thrive in school.

1.3.5 Special Educational Needs and Disabilities (SEND) in Crisis

Children requiring specialised interventions, whether for autism spectrum disorders, learning disabilities, or emotional and behavioural difficulties, were disproportionately affected by local authority budget cuts of 17% or more (9). Longer waits for assessment and reduced access to trained professionals left a generation of pupils lacking the tailored support they needed. In some regions, cuts were even more dramatic, with the North West facing a 22% reduction in SEND provision (9).

The downstream effect on schools—particularly those already struggling with large class sizes—was profound. Teachers and assistants in deprived areas could not provide the level of attention or resources needed for high-needs pupils, leading to further exclusion, absenteeism, or a decline in overall academic performance. For these students, the education system became less an engine of opportunity and more a site of repeated frustration and marginalisation, paving the way for poorer health and social outcomes in adulthood.

1.4 A Fractured System Meets a Global Crisis: The Impact of COVID-19

1.4.1 Unprecedented School Closures

The COVID-19 pandemic triggered a historic disruption: as of March 2020, 1.6 billion children globally were out of school (10). In the UK, roughly 99% of pupils were locked out of classrooms (11). While the stated purpose was to curtail viral transmission, subsequent epidemiological analyses indicated that school closures had uncertain or negligible impacts on infection rates (12,13). Nonetheless, the policy decision to close schools for extended periods became a defining feature of the early pandemic response.

For children in well-resourced families, remote learning—while not ideal—remained feasible through private tutoring, stable internet connections, dedicated study areas, and parental oversight. For those already disadvantaged by austerity-era cuts, the experience was far more devastating. Students lacked laptops or tablets, families could not afford consistent broadband, and overcrowded living conditions offered no quiet study space.

1.4.2   The Digital Divide

As schools pivoted to online instruction, the term "digital divide" became emblematic of educational inequalities. In the UK, approximately 27% of the poorest households had no suitable device for remote learning; many also lacked a reliable internet connection (14,15). Even when the government pledged to distribute laptops, supply chain issues and administrative hurdles left numerous families waiting for weeks or months.

Data from the Education Policy Institute revealed that only 38% of state school students enjoyed a full remote school day during the first lockdown, compared to 74% of private school students (14). This discrepancy reflected more than just device shortages: it encompassed differences in teacher-student ratios, the capacity of teachers to conduct live lessons, and the resilience of school leadership teams under pandemic pressures. As a result, children who were already behind before the pandemic now risked falling irrecoverably further behind.

1.4.3   Private Tutoring and the Escalation of Inequality

A parallel trend was the sharp uptick in private tutoring. Wealthier families turned to online tuition services to fill the gap left by schools in lockdown, effectively customising children's learning experiences. Disadvantaged pupils, by contrast, relied largely on whatever minimal provision their schools could offer. Overstretched teachers, sometimes managing their own childcare at home, could not replicate the intensity or individualisation of private tutoring.

The result? A significant academic chasm, as wealthier students made steady progress, while disadvantaged students stagnated or regressed. By the time schools reopened, many researchers estimated that the poverty-related gap in achievement had widened by at least 4.7 months (14,16). In effect, the pandemic lockdowns acted as an accelerator of pre-existing educational disparities, setting the stage for a further widening of health inequalities down the line.

1.4.4   School Closures and Social Support Systems

Critically, schools do far more than impart academic instruction. They serve as sites of nutritional support, mental health referrals, safeguarding against domestic violence, and consistent adult supervision for at-risk children.

During closures, these safety nets dissolved. Many children lost access to free school meals—often their main source of balanced nutrition—while parents faced income and job insecurity (17).

Such disruptions in routine exacerbated stress within households, amplifying the risk of adverse childhood experiences that can have enduring psychological and physiological impacts. For those already living in poverty, the combined effect of losing out on learning, school meals, and emotional support created a crisis of compounding vulnerabilities (1). Post-traumatic stress, heightened anxiety, and social isolation threatened to derail development at a critical juncture, with implications for children's longer-term mental and physical health.

1.4.5 Reopening Schools: Enduring Funding Disparities

When schools eventually reopened, the pre-existing funding differentials persisted and, in some cases, deepened. Data suggested that per-pupil spending in the most deprived schools declined by 14%, compared with 9% in the least deprived (8). In practice, this meant fewer resources to address the complex educational and emotional repercussions of the pandemic. Small-group catch-up tutoring, for instance, remained sporadic, dependent on inconsistent or delayed government grants.

Meanwhile, communities that had lost youth clubs, early intervention services, and family support programmes during austerity were left attempting to rebuild fragile support infrastructures under extraordinary conditions. Far from galvanising a robust, equitable policy response, the pandemic's aftermath frequently led to piecemeal solutions—further entrenching the notion that educational recovery would depend on local-level improvisation rather than systematic, nationwide reform.

1.5   Consequences Across the Life Course: Health, Well-Being, and Opportunity

1.5.1   Learning Loss and Long-Term Outcomes

Learning loss in childhood ripples throughout the life course. Evidence indicates that children who fail to develop strong literacy and numeracy skills by the end of primary school are more likely to fall behind in secondary education and face reduced employability in adult life (17). The COVID-19 disruptions, layered atop austerity-era funding cuts, place a generation at risk of suboptimal qualifications, lower lifetime earnings, and precarious employment.

Research on the link between education and health unequivocally shows that adults with less schooling experience disproportionately higher rates of cardiovascular disease, obesity, mental health issues, and cigarette smoking (2,3). Even modest reductions in average years of schooling at a population level can lead to significant hikes in all-cause mortality and years of life lost (18). By cutting short the education of disadvantaged children, the system effectively primes them for poorer health trajectories, with associated burdens on the NHS and social services.

1.5.2   *Psychosocial Implications and Toxic Stress*

Children from low-income backgrounds often experience a range of psychosocial stressors, including housing insecurity, food insecurity, and exposure to neighbourhood violence. Effective schooling can serve as a buffer by providing structure, mentorship, and respite. When schooling itself becomes a source of stress—due to resource scarcity, negative peer dynamics, or inadequate support for special needs—its protective effect erodes.

The pandemic introduced new layers of uncertainty, with lockdowns, potential bereavement, and financial upheaval all intensifying mental health strain. Students who had tenuous connections to school pre-pandemic were at heightened risk of disengagement, isolation, and an ongoing sense of hopelessness (1). Over time, these feelings can accumulate into "toxic stress", harming the developing brain's architecture, weakening immune function, and worsening long-term health outcomes.

1.5.3   *Intergenerational Cycles of Disadvantage*

Children who exit adolescence with poor qualifications are more likely to have limited earning potential and less stable employment, feeding into a repeating cycle of disadvantage. As parents, they may struggle to provide adequately for their own children, reinforcing the conditions that perpetuate underachievement. From a macro perspective, these cyclical patterns hamper community cohesion, reinforce geographic pockets of deprivation, and exacerbate wealth and health gaps nationally.

Moreover, mounting evidence suggests that the "COVID generation"—those whose schooling was severely disrupted—may experience compounded setbacks as they transition into adulthood. Reduced readiness for higher education or vocational training will likely yield a generation whose health vulnerabilities reflect the accumulated scarring of multiple crises: austerity, pandemic-driven learning loss, and the cost-of-living shocks that followed.

1.6   International Comparisons and Lessons Learned

1.6.1   *Educational Inequalities on the Global Stage*

The UK is not alone in grappling with pandemic-induced educational setbacks; however, the entrenched disparities produced by austerity placed it at a disadvantage compared to certain European counterparts. Nations with robust, well-funded social infrastructures—where child poverty rates were lower and digital access was more universal—navigated remote learning with comparatively less educational loss.

For instance, countries like Denmark managed shorter school closures, quicker transitions to hybrid models, and strong local authority engagement to ensure that vulnerable children were reached (10). By contrast, in the UK, inconsistencies in government guidance, delayed technology rollouts, and existing socioeconomic schisms led to a more pronounced academic and digital divide.

1.6.2 The Link to Health Systems and Social Policy

Cross-national studies of the pandemic highlight how countries that align educational policies with broader social supports—universal childcare, comprehensive school meal programmes, accessible mental health services—tend to preserve a greater degree of equity. This alignment mitigates the worst health repercussions of educational interruptions. In the UK, however, austerity had already weakened these complementary safety nets.

Comparative analyses also indicate that where health and education ministries collaborate in formulating crisis responses (e.g., distributing hygiene kits, co-locating testing facilities in schools, providing mental health hotlines for students), disruptions can be more effectively managed (1). Such strategies, which emphasise integrated service delivery, may help buffer children from educational trauma and associated health declines.

1.7 Charting a Post-Pandemic Path Forward

1.7.1 Addressing Digital Inequity

Any meaningful post-pandemic strategy must tackle the digital divide. Universal internet access, funding for devices, and training for educators in digital pedagogy can lay the groundwork for more equitable remote or blended learning models in the future. More ambitious proposals might posit that internet connectivity should be treated as a utility akin to water or electricity—essential for modern life.

Ensuring that children from deprived backgrounds are not further marginalised by technological deficits requires not only governmental resource allocation but also partnerships with private tech companies and non-profit organisations. The aim is to build resilience in the education system so that subsequent emergencies—be they localised school closures or national crises—do not disproportionately harm the poorest students.

1.7.2 *Strengthening the Early Years*

Substantial evidence indicates that interventions in early childhood yield the highest returns on investment, both in academic achievement and in health outcomes (8). Reinstating or expanding children's centres, boosting funding for nursery places, and providing targeted family support can help close developmental gaps before children even enter primary school.

These measures should be coupled with robust home-visiting programmes and parental engagement strategies. By equipping parents with knowledge and resources—from nutrition guidance to literacy tools—early childhood services can serve as a bulwark against the cascading disadvantages that define so many children's formative years.

1.7.3 *Equitable Funding and School Infrastructure*

A radical rethinking of the school funding formula could direct a higher weighting of resources towards areas of high deprivation, reversing the trends under austerity. Teachers in underfunded schools should receive enhanced support to reduce class sizes, increase access to professional development, and bolster mental health services for pupils.

Short-term catch-up funding, while useful, cannot substitute for systemic reform. Policymakers could consider ring-fenced budgets for SEND provision, ensuring that waiting lists and service gaps do not continue to penalise children with additional needs. Additionally, frameworks that prioritise mental health and well-being—such as on-site counsellors or partnerships with child psychologists—can help reclaim schools as supportive, community-focused spaces.

1.7.4 *Holistic Child Poverty Interventions*

Addressing the educational divide necessitates broader anti-poverty strategies. Adequate welfare benefits, fair wage standards, stable housing policies, and affordable childcare collectively underpin a child's capacity to succeed in school. Linking social protection programmes to school attendance and performance can incentivise families and remove barriers, but only if these programmes are designed with dignity, accessibility, and robust funding in mind.

Policy alignment is critical: initiatives that improve maternal health, reduce food insecurity, and enable parental employment all feed into better educational outcomes for children. Governments serious about bridging the attainment gap might consider adopting a "Health in All Policies" approach, integrating health and education objectives at every stage of policymaking—recognising that deprived communities often require multi-faceted interventions to ameliorate cyclical disadvantage.

1.7.5 Capitalising on Community and Grassroots Movements

The pandemic period saw the rise of grassroots, volunteer-led efforts to support children's learning—ranging from laptop donation drives to community homework clubs. Harnessing this local energy can be part of a comprehensive solution. Community-led initiatives often prove agile in addressing gaps that formal systems struggle to fill, especially in reaching families wary of official agencies. Local authorities, schools, and civil society groups could formalise partnerships to coordinate resources. For instance, libraries or community centres might function as hub sites for device loans, tutoring, and nutritious meal programmes. While such grassroots endeavours cannot single-handedly rectify systemic underinvestment, they can serve as a crucial supplement—especially when properly funded and integrated into regional and national strategies.

1.8 Conclusion

Education is at once a bulwark and a beacon: it protects children from the pitfalls of poverty and guides them towards healthier, more fulfilling lives. In Britain, both the protective and liberating aspects of education have been undermined by a decade of austerity, which drastically reduced funding in the very communities that most needed robust, comprehensive schooling. The COVID-19 pandemic then laid bare these inequities, deepening them at an alarming rate.

Far from being a neutral crisis, the pandemic acted as an accelerant of existing structural fault lines. Disadvantaged children were locked out of remote learning, denied private tutoring, and severed from vital services ordinarily accessed through schools. The attainment gap—already measured in months—expanded into a yawning chasm. This educational emergency, in turn, presages a generational health crisis, as inadequate schooling fosters higher rates of chronic illness, reduced life expectancy, and poorer mental health over the life course.

Addressing these challenges demands more than piecemeal catch-up efforts. It calls for a wholesale reimagining of how education is financed and delivered, particularly to those who have historically been left behind. Early childhood interventions, digital equity, and integrated social support systems must converge to form a coherent, future-proof strategy. If policymakers, educators, and communities can unite around the imperative of reducing educational inequalities, the dividends will be far-reaching—improved social mobility, healthier citizens, and a more resilient society. Conversely, if the lessons of austerity and the pandemic go unheeded, Britain risks entrenching a new underclass of children whose prospects remain tragically tethered to their postcode and parental income. The stakes could not be higher: every child's right to learn is, ultimately, a right to health, dignity, and a life unbounded by the inequalities of the past.

References

1. Hayre, J. COVID-19, education and child health. BMJ Paediatr Open. 2023;7(1):e001863.
2. Khan N, Javed Z, Acquah I, Hagan K, Khan M, Valero-Elizondo J, et al. Low educational attainment is associated with higher all-cause and cardiovascular mortality in the United States adult population. BMC Public Health. 2023;23(1):900.
3. Gilman SE, Martin LT, Abrams DB, Kawachi I, Kubzansky L, Loucks EB, et al. Educational attainment and cigarette smoking: a causal association? Int J Epidemiol. 2008;37(3):615–24.
4. Borgonovi F, Pokropek A. Education and self-reported health: evidence from 23 countries on the role of years of schooling, cognitive skills and social capital. PLoS One. 2016;11(2):e0149716.
5. Courtin E, Nafilyan V, Glymour M, Goldberg M, Berr C, Berkman LF, et al. Long-term effects of compulsory schooling on physical, mental and cognitive ageing: a natural experiment. J Epidemiol Community Health. 2019;73(4):370–6.
6. Department for Education. School funding in England, 2010–11 to 2020–21: experimental official statistics. London: DfE; 2020.
7. Sibieta L, Farquharson C, Waltmann B, Tahir I. 2021 annual report on education spending in England. London: The Institute for Fiscal Studies; 2021.
8. Education Policy Institute. Education in England: annual report 2019. London: EPI; 2019.
9. Parveen N. Funding for pupils with special educational needs drops 17%. The Guardian. 2019 Apr 4.
10. McKinsey & Company. Coronavirus shut down schools worldwide. McKinsey & Company; 2020.
11. Whittaker F. Coronavirus: school attendance around 1%, finds DfE analysis. Schools Week. 2020.
12. Fukumoto K, McClean CT, Nakagawa K. No causal effect of school closures in Japan on the spread of COVID-19 in Spring 2020. Nat Med. 2021;27(12):2111–9.
13. Lewis SJ, Munro APS, Smith GD, Pollock AM. Closing schools is not evidence based and harms children. BMJ. 2021;372:n521.
14. Hutchinson J, Reader M, Akhal A. Education in England: annual report 2020. Education Policy Institute; 2020.
15. Gilhooly R. How lockdown has affected children's lives at home. Children's Commissioner; 2020.
16. Andrew A, Cattan S, Costa Dias M, Farquharson C, Kraftman L, Krutikova S, et al. Educational gaps are growing during lockdown. The Institute for Fiscal Studies; 2020.

17. Centre for Global Development. Learning loss and student dropouts during the COVID-19 pandemic: a review of the evidence two years after schools shut down. Washington (DC): CGDev; 2022.
18. Christakis DA, Van Cleve W, Zimmerman FJ. Estimation of US children's educational attainment and years of life lost associated with primary school closures during the coronavirus disease 2019 pandemic. JAMA Netw Open. 2020;3(11):e2028786.

2 Food Exclusivity and Insecurity

Introduction

Food, at its core, is more than mere sustenance: it is a powerful determinant of health, educational outcomes, socioeconomic opportunities, and overall life trajectory. In childhood, this significance is heightened dramatically. The early years—especially the first 1,000 days from conception to a child's second birthday—represent a golden window in which adequate nutrition exerts an outsized influence on brain architecture, organ formation, and immune strength. Deficiencies or imbalances during this crucial phase can precipitate lifelong, often irreversible, impairments in cognitive functioning, growth, and morbidity patterns. Yet the nutritional needs of a child do not end abruptly after toddlerhood; rather, they continue through adolescence and beyond, shaping physical, cognitive, and emotional well-being at every developmental stage.

In modern Britain, food insecurity has grown into a pervasive public health challenge—a reality starkly reflected in the rising demand for food banks, the prevalence of childhood obesity, and the disparate nutritional outcomes observed across different socioeconomic groups. This phenomenon was exacerbated by two major upheavals: first, the period of austerity between 2010 and 2019, during which social safety nets were severely strained; and second, the COVID-19 pandemic, which magnified existing inequalities and pushed numerous families to the brink. This chapter delves into the nexus of childhood nutrition and social inequity, examining the interplay between austerity policies, food insecurity, obesity, and broader health outcomes. Through a life course perspective, it highlights the profound, long-term repercussions of inadequate or imbalanced nutrition on individuals and societies.

In weaving together these strands, the chapter aims not only to provide a critical understanding of how food insecurity and nutritional exclusivity undermine children's health and potential but also to illustrate how these vulnerabilities were laid bare by the COVID-19 pandemic. In the face of this crisis, the urgency of addressing systemic deficiencies—be they in welfare provision, community support structures, or educational policies—has

DOI: 10.4324/9781003312529-3

become inescapable. As Britain endeavours to rebuild, ensuring equitable access to nutritious food for all children stands as one of the most pressing moral and economic imperatives.

2.1 Conceptual Foundations: Food Insecurity, Nutritional Inequity, and Child Health

2.1.1 Defining Food Insecurity

Food insecurity is broadly defined as the inability of households to secure adequate food, in both quality and quantity, to meet the dietary needs of all members (1). However, this definition masks the manifold dimensions of the problem: questions of cultural acceptability, the psychological stress of uncertain food supply, and the nutritional sufficiency of the food consumed. In the British context, food insecurity has evolved in tandem with market forces, welfare reforms, and changing social norms. It is often manifested in a reliance on food banks, skipping meals, or substituting healthier options for cheaper, calorie-dense but nutrient-poor alternatives (2).

Such substitutions form the backbone of "food exclusivity", wherein nutritionally rich foods like fruits, vegetables, and lean proteins are priced out of the reach of low-income households (3). Rather than simply lacking food, families find themselves restricted to a narrower selection of inexpensive but nutrient-poor fare—often laden with saturated fats, refined carbohydrates, and added sugars. This dual phenomenon of "overfed but undernourished" underscores the modern paradox: obesity rates and micronutrient deficiencies frequently coexist within the same individual, household, or community (4).

2.1.2 Nutrition in Early Childhood and the First 1,000 Days

The significance of nutrition in the first 1,000 days—from conception to age two—cannot be overstated. Adequate maternal nutrition during pregnancy supports foetal growth and reduces the risk of intrauterine growth restriction (IUGR), which can precipitate low birth weight and neonatal complications (5). During infancy, exclusive breastfeeding for the first six months—recommended by the World Health Organization—contributes to optimal neurodevelopment and immunological resilience (6). Complementary feeding thereafter, if balanced and age-appropriate, cements the foundations for lifelong eating habits and metabolic functioning.

Deficiencies that arise during this critical window may result in stunting, impaired cognitive development, and weakened immunity, creating a ripple effect felt well into adolescence and adulthood (7). For instance, iron deficiency anaemia in infancy can lead to delayed myelination in the brain, disrupting processes crucial for memory and learning (8). Similarly, inadequate vitamin D intake hinders bone mineralisation, raising the risk of rickets and future osteopenia (9). The immediate and cumulative costs of such deficiencies are enormous, not only for the individual child but also for the wider society through increased healthcare expenditure and diminished human capital.

2.1.3 Beyond the Early Years: The Ongoing Relevance of Nutritional Adequacy

While the first 1,000 days are essential, nutrition remains critical throughout childhood and adolescence. Rapid periods of growth—particularly in adolescence—demand heightened intakes of micronutrients, such as iron, calcium, and zinc, as well as macronutrients balanced in protein, carbohydrates, and healthy fats (10). Simultaneously, the educational and social expectations intensify: children require sufficient cognitive resources to engage in complex learning, problem-solving, and emotional regulation (11). When nutritional needs remain unmet, academic performance, physical fitness, and mental well-being can all deteriorate.

Importantly, the emergence of childhood obesity represents a complex manifestation of malnutrition (12). Obesity's roots lie in the interplay between dietary habits, physical activity, genetic predisposition, and socioeconomic factors. In low-income settings, energy-dense, low-quality food is often cheaper and more accessible than nutrient-rich alternatives. This accessibility gap contributes to a higher incidence of overweight and obesity in disadvantaged communities, reflecting how inequalities in purchasing power translate directly into health outcomes (13).

2.2 The Socio-Political Backdrop: Austerity and Its Legacy

2.2.1 Austerity Measures (2010–2019) and Their Implications

Between 2010 and 2019, the UK government undertook extensive austerity measures aimed at reducing public spending and curtailing the national deficit. While proponents argued that fiscal responsibility was necessary following the global financial crisis, the ramifications for social welfare, child services, and public health were profound (14). An estimated £30 billion in cuts to social security contributed to the erosion of living standards for many households already at the margins. Benefit freezes, sanctions, and the so-called "bedroom tax" (spare room subsidy) magnified economic hardships, leaving families struggling to cover housing, utilities, and food costs (15).

For children, the aftermath was acutely felt in the rise of food insecurity and malnutrition. Households with diminished purchasing power gravitated towards cheaper, nutrient-poor foods, resulting in inadequate dietary diversity and higher obesity rates (16). Simultaneously, local authorities—whose budgets were severely squeezed—found themselves unable to sustain many community-based interventions designed to cushion vulnerable families. Holiday breakfast clubs, youth clubs, and after-school programmes that once alleviated food and childcare pressures faced funding cuts or complete closure, compounding the crisis (17).

2.2.2   Food Bank Usage as a Barometer of Crisis

Few indicators illustrate the depth of Britain's food insecurity during this period as starkly as the explosion in food bank usage. The Trussell Trust, which operates around two-thirds of the country's food banks, distributed approximately 40,000 three-day emergency food parcels in 2010–2011, a number that leapt to over 1.6 million by 2018–2019 (18). Independent food aid providers, similarly, reported exponential growth in demand. This trend not only signalled deteriorating household income but also underscored broader structural failures in the social safety net.

Parents forced to choose between rent, utilities, and groceries increasingly turned to emergency provisions, highlighting the precarious balance many families maintained even before an unforeseen expense or a reduction in working hours (19). Stigma, meanwhile, discouraged some families from seeking help, suggesting that recorded data might underestimate the true scale of deprivation (20). For children reliant on these parcels, the nutritional composition—often non-perishable, tinned, or processed foods—was generally less balanced than an ideal diet. Consequently, food banks themselves became caught in a conundrum: how to offer nutritionally appropriate options amidst limited resources and the necessity of shelf-stable products (21).

2.2.3   The Exclusive Cost of Healthy Eating

A major driver of food insecurity is the cost differential between healthy and less healthy foods. One study found that, between 2002 and 2012, prices for fruit and vegetables rose by 35%, while the cost of sugary and fatty foods remained relatively stable (22). By 2012, purchasing 1,000 kilocalories of healthy food (e.g., whole grains, lean proteins, and fresh produce) was nearly three times more expensive than equivalent calories of highly processed items (23). This "food exclusivity" effectively locked low-income families out of healthier diets, fuelling a vicious cycle of nutrient deficiencies and obesity.

As austerity took hold, these cost disparities sharpened. Families already spending a large share of disposable income on housing found it increasingly difficult to sustain balanced diets (24). The policy impetus emphasising personal responsibility and food budgeting tips—e.g., "buy in bulk", "choose cheaper cuts of meat"—overlooked the structural reality of precarious employment, debt, and limited cooking facilities that many families faced. The net result was a generation of children who, even if not clinically underweight, were consistently missing out on essential micronutrients (25).

2.3   Nutritional Deficits and Consequences for Child Development

2.3.1   Cognitive and Educational Implications

The links between childhood nutrition and cognition are direct and profound. Children experiencing chronic undernutrition—whether measured in stunting, anaemia, or overall dietary quality—tend to display lower academic achievement, reduced attention spans, and diminished cognitive flexibility (26). Even mild iron deficiency can hamper neurotransmitter function, impairing concentration, and working memory (27). Such impediments often manifest in poorer literacy, numeracy, and problem-solving skills, perpetuating cycles of disadvantage that extend beyond schooling into adulthood.

Furthermore, children going to school hungry face immediate disadvantages: difficulty focusing, irritability, and decreased motivation (28). Teachers report that hungry pupils are more likely to exhibit behavioural issues and less likely to engage in class activities or form positive peer relationships (29). The interplay of hunger, stress, and shame can compound, as children internalise stigma or experience bullying, further eroding self-esteem and academic performance.

2.3.2   Physical Health Risks

Nutritional adequacy in childhood is fundamental for preventing both undernutrition and overnutrition. On one end of the spectrum, chronic undernutrition manifests as stunting, low body weight, and susceptibility to infections due to compromised immunity (30). On the other end, high rates of childhood overweight and obesity, commonly seen in low-income communities, amplify the risk of early-onset non-communicable diseases such as type 2 diabetes, cardiovascular disease, and certain cancers (31). This dual burden is increasingly visible in Britain, reflecting a pattern once primarily associated with developing countries undergoing rapid nutrition transitions.

Evidence suggests that malnutrition in childhood—be it under- or overnutrition—paves the way for adverse health outcomes in adulthood. Stunted children often become stunted adults, facing reduced work capacity and increased morbidity (32). Overweight children frequently progress to become overweight adults, with a heightened risk of metabolic syndrome, musculoskeletal disorders, and psychological issues (33). From a policy standpoint, addressing these extremes of malnutrition through measures that ensure access to balanced diets is crucial for breaking intergenerational cycles of poor health.

2.3.3 Psychosocial and Emotional Well-being

Food insecurity is not purely a matter of physical health. It also exerts a profound psychological toll on children, who may sense familial distress, worry about where their next meal is coming from, and absorb the stigma of poverty (34). Chronic stress linked to uncertain food supplies can alter the developing brain's architecture, particularly in regions governing emotional regulation and executive function (35). This stress can predispose children to anxiety and depressive disorders, impairing social relationships and decreasing resilience.

Adolescents, too, are vulnerable to these psychosocial pressures. Body image anxieties intersect with issues of dietary quality and family resources. For instance, teenagers in food-insecure households may skip meals or adopt disordered eating habits to help manage scarce food supplies, potentially fuelling eating disorders over time (36). While obesity remains a key public health concern, the psychological drivers and outcomes of weight gain in deprived contexts must be recognised as deeply entwined with issues of trauma, stress, and low self-efficacy.

2.4 Food Insecurity in the Context of the COVID-19 Pandemic

2.4.1 The Magnification of Existing Inequalities

The COVID-19 pandemic, declared in March 2020, arrived against an already precarious backdrop of food insecurity and child malnutrition. As lockdowns closed schools and workplaces, families reliant on free school meals or part-time wages lost critical forms of support almost overnight (37). Food bank demand surged—by mid-2020, the Trussell Trust reported an 89% increase in requests compared to the same period the previous year (38). This reflected not only an upturn in job losses and furloughs but also the fragility of household finances following a decade of welfare cuts.

School closures robbed many children of their sole reliable daily meal, intensifying nutritional deficits and placing additional strains on parents (39). Though the UK government introduced voucher schemes and free school meal replacements, inconsistent delivery and administrative barriers hindered the reach and effectiveness of these programmes (40). For undocumented or marginalised families, fears of data-sharing and deportation further dissuaded participation in publicly funded support schemes (41).

2.4.2   Disruptions to the Food Supply Chain

The pandemic also disrupted food supply chains, with panic buying, price inflation, and stock shortages disproportionately affecting low-income households (42). Reduced supermarket hours or online shopping requirements disadvantaged those without reliable transportation, internet access, or sufficient funds to bulk buy. Many families who had not previously experienced food insecurity suddenly found themselves in need, placing additional pressure on community-level food initiatives (43).

Children confined to inadequate living spaces, often with limited or no outdoor access, faced heightened risks of inactivity and stress-eating, which could exacerbate obesity trends (44). Conversely, families wholly reliant on rapidly dwindling community support might have skipped meals or reduced portion sizes, exacerbating undernutrition. These polarised experiences underscored the complexity and diversity of food insecurity's manifestations during the pandemic.

2.4.3   Digital Divide and Educational Setbacks

A less visible but significant impact of COVID-19 on child nutrition was the "digital divide". With schooling shifted online, children lacking reliable internet or digital devices were cut off from virtual lessons, online resources, and interactions with peers. In many cases, these same households grappled with food insecurity, forming a nexus of disadvantage (45). Without regular school lunches, teacher oversight, and extracurricular support, children from food-insecure households experienced academic setbacks, diminished socialisation, and an exacerbated sense of marginalisation (46).

In some communities, charitable organisations, faith groups, and local volunteers filled the gaps, offering meal deliveries and laptop donations. Yet these efforts, commendable as they were, could not substitute for systemic, well-funded interventions. The risk of a "lost generation"—children whose foundational years were marked by nutritional deficiencies, academic disruptions, and psychosocial strain—loomed large (47).

2.5   A Life Course Perspective: Long-Term Implications of Food Exclusivity and Insecurity

2.5.1   Early-Life Nutritional Deficits and Adult Health Outcomes

The life course approach emphasises that nutritional insults during childhood cast a long shadow over adulthood. Inadequate macro- and micronutrient intake can impair organ formation, hamper immune maturity, and perpetuate metabolic disorders that only manifest later in life (48). The phenomenon known as the "foetal origins of adult disease" highlights how adverse conditions in utero contribute to raised risks of hypertension, type 2 diabetes, and coronary artery disease in adulthood (49). When compounded by sub-optimal nutrition in early childhood and adolescence, these risks intensify, shaping an adult population burdened by chronic illnesses.

In Britain, austerity and pandemic-era pressures have likely birthed a cohort of children with heightened vulnerability to a range of non-communicable diseases. From a public health standpoint, ignoring these early-stage ineq-uities invites significant future costs, both financially (through healthcare expenditure) and socially (through lost productivity and deepened inequali-ties) (50). Strategic investments in childhood nutrition thus represent not only a moral obligation but also a pragmatic approach to mitigating the long-range burden of disease.

2.5.2 *Intergenerational Cycles of Poverty and Malnutrition*

Food insecurity entrenches cycles of poverty and ill-health that extend across generations. Children who grow up malnourished tend to have poorer educa-tional attainment, reduced employment prospects, and lower lifetime earn-ings, perpetuating the very conditions that fuel food insecurity (51). This cyclical dynamic is evident in Britain's most deprived areas, where poverty, inadequate housing, and under-resourced schools converge to stifle upwards social mobility.

Moreover, young people who enter adulthood with chronic health condi-tions or psychological disturbances rooted in poor nutrition may struggle to break out of disadvantaged labour markets. As parents, they may lack the resources to provide nutritionally adequate diets for their own children, thus perpetuating the cycle (52). Breaking this intergenerational chain requires comprehensive social policies that address not only immediate nutritional needs but also the structural determinants of poverty.

2.5.3 *Societal and Economic Burdens*

A nutritionally compromised childhood yields steep societal costs—ranging from spiralling healthcare expenses to weakened labour force participa-tion. Estimations suggest that malnutrition and obesity together cost the NHS billions each year in treatment for related conditions (53). However, these figures do not fully account for indirect losses in productivity, social care demands, and reduced quality of life.

Wider economic analyses, such as those aligned with the "social deter-minants of health" framework, repeatedly highlight that policy intervention targeting child nutrition offer robust returns on investment (54). Improving food security alleviates financial strain on healthcare systems, heightens educational outcomes, and fosters a healthier, more productive workforce.

As Britain grapples with post-pandemic recovery, failing to address child nutrition could amount to a missed opportunity for bolstering socioeconomic resilience.

2.6   Policy Responses and Gaps: Before, During, and Beyond COVID-19

2.6.1   Pre-Pandemic Measures

Before COVID-19, Britain had some noteworthy anti-hunger and child nutrition initiatives, including free school meals, the Healthy Start scheme for pregnant women and families with young children, and local authority-led breakfast clubs (55). However, the widespread impact of austerity often negated these efforts: real-term cuts to local authority budgets forced many programmes to scale back or shut down. Eligibility criteria for free school meals frequently excluded struggling families, including those with irregular immigration status or just above income thresholds (56).

The Homelessness Reduction Act 2017 and various local welfare assistance schemes indirectly influenced household food security by providing limited support to families in crisis (57). Yet these initiatives did not tackle the broader structural challenges, such as the high cost of living relative to wages, precarious employment, or inflated housing markets. In short, pre-pandemic policies, while beneficial to some, fell short of a holistic approach that could shield children from the nexus of food insecurity and poverty.

2.6.2   Pandemic-Era Responses: Successes and Shortcomings

Once COVID-19 took hold, the Government moved swiftly to introduce schemes such as the Coronavirus Job Retention Scheme (furlough) and the COVID Winter Grant to mitigate income loss (58). Specific to child nutrition, a voucher system was launched for those eligible for free school meals. These measures undoubtedly prevented a worse humanitarian crisis; however, significant administrative and logistical flaws were evident—vouchers sometimes failed to arrive, were restricted to certain supermarkets, or could not be used for online shopping (59).

Furthermore, the digital and socio-cultural barriers meant many eligible families remained unaware of or reluctant to access such support (41). Child poverty campaigners, including high-profile figures, repeatedly urged the Government to extend free school meals through holiday periods; a measure that was eventually implemented in fits and starts (60). The patchwork nature of these interventions highlights how, without cohesive, long-term policy frameworks, crises merely exacerbate existing inequalities.

2.6.3 Opportunities for Post-Pandemic Reform

The tumult of the pandemic has arguably triggered a moment of collective reckoning. Public discourse increasingly recognises that food insecurity is a systemic issue requiring sustained intervention. Potential reform avenues include:

1. Expanding Free School Meals: Lowering the income threshold and ensuring all families in need can access school-based nutrition, regardless of immigration status. Universal free school meals at primary the level are also advocated by some experts to reduce stigma and administrative hurdles (61).
2. Strengthening Healthy Start and Related Schemes: Raising the value of vouchers, broadening eligibility, and simplifying the application process can promote improved maternal and child nutrition (62). Digitalising vouchers while preserving an option for offline use may also lessen barriers.
3. Tackling the Cost of Healthy Food: Introducing subsidies or price regulations for nutritious staples—fruit, vegetables, whole grains—could narrow the affordability gap. Taxation of ultra-processed foods or sugar-sweetened beverages might funnel revenue into food poverty interventions (63).
4. Integrating Nutrition into Broader Social Policies: Linking housing, employment, and welfare reforms to nutritional objectives ensures that families can maintain stable incomes and living situations conducive to healthy eating (64).
5. Investing in Community Infrastructure: Local authorities require adequate funding to rejuvenate youth clubs, breakfast clubs, and holiday provision schemes—spaces where children can receive both nourishing meals and social support (17). Place-based interventions that empower communities to grow their own produce (e.g., allotments and community gardens) can also enhance food resilience.

2.7 Grassroots, Community Action, and the Role of Civil Society

2.7.1 Food Banks, Social Supermarkets, and Mutual Aid

Amidst government retrenchment, voluntary groups, and community organisations have played a pivotal role in alleviating child hunger. Food banks, while never intended as a permanent fixture, offer emergency relief and have become essential community anchors (65). Newer models, such as social supermarkets and community pantries, aim to provide discounted groceries in a dignified setting, sometimes paired with financial counselling or job support (66). Mutual aid groups, especially during COVID-19, sprang up to organise meal deliveries, grocery shopping for vulnerable neighbours, and signposting to available services (67). Though crucial for short-term relief, these grassroots interventions acknowledge the need for systemic policy change to address root causes.

2.7.2   *Stigma, Dignity, and Empowerment*

Central to any localised or civil society initiative is the issue of stigma. Families facing food insecurity may feel ashamed to seek help, especially if they perceive a social judgement or lack of empathy from authorities. Consequently, initiatives that foreground dignity—where users contribute financially at a reduced rate or volunteer in exchange—often see higher uptake (68). School-based breakfast clubs open to all pupils, irrespective of income, reduce the stigma of means-tested provision and can foster a stronger sense of community ownership (69).

Moreover, empowering parents and caregivers with nutrition literacy, budgeting skills, and cooking workshops can boost self-reliance, provided these strategies do not drift into "victim-blaming" narratives that ignore structural inequities (70). Hence, the most successful community interventions strike a balance between immediate relief, capacity-building, and advocacy for broader reforms.

2.7.3   *Advocating for Policy Change*

Civil society organisations and academics increasingly collaborate to push for evidence-based policy. Examples include forging alliances with healthcare professionals, educators, and child psychologists to spotlight how malnutrition undercuts educational attainment and long-term well-being (71). Campaigns run by sports personalities and charities have spurred wider public debate, revealing an emerging consensus that childhood food insecurity is not an inevitability but a solvable crisis (72). Legislative proposals, such as extending free school meals to all families receiving Universal Credit, are a testament to this sustained advocacy (73).

2.8   Conclusion: Charting a Path Towards Nutritional Equity

Food is the bedrock upon which a child's immediate well-being and future prosperity are constructed. This holds true from the prenatal phase through adolescence, where balanced nutrition underpins everything from organ formation and immune competence to cognitive function and emotional regulation. In Britain, austerity-era social welfare contractions exposed and exacerbated existing vulnerabilities, catapulting food insecurity to unprecedented levels.

Although temporary measures—whether Government-led or grassroots—have mitigated some of the worst effects, structural challenges persist. Families continue to face trade-offs between housing costs and grocery bills, healthy foods remain comparatively expensive, and children from deprived backgrounds bear the brunt of these inequities in the form of malnutrition, obesity, and stifled opportunities.

The COVID-19 pandemic served as both a magnifier of these issues and a potential catalyst for change. School closures, widespread unemployment, and disrupted food supply chains laid bare the fragility of the current system. Yet they also galvanised community action and intensified public discourse around the urgent need for more inclusive, robust policies. What emerges is a dual imperative: to address the immediate hunger and nutritional deficits afflicting children today, and to enact long-term structural reforms that ensure equitable access to healthy food for generations to come.

In this light, the policy conversation must go beyond emergency aid and short-term fixes. It calls for investing in comprehensive anti-poverty measures, strengthening the social security net, subsidising healthy foods, and fostering inclusive community spaces. It demands a concerted effort to dismantle the stigma surrounding food aid and to empower families through education, participation, and advocacy. Above all, it requires recognition that child nutrition is an investment in the nation's future. Failure to safeguard children's nutritional well-being now virtually guarantees heightened healthcare costs, reduced economic productivity, and entrenched social inequalities down the line.

As the UK transitions out of the pandemic's immediate crisis, policymakers, practitioners, and civil society alike face a watershed moment. With sustained political will, targeted funding, and evidence-driven interventions, Britain can begin to rewrite its narrative on child hunger and malnutrition. The goal is both urgent and achievable: a society in which no child's potential is sacrificed to the fortunes of postcode or parental income, and where food insecurity is relegated to a historical footnote rather than a persistent social indictment.

References

1. Food and Agriculture Organization (FAO). The state of food security and nutrition in the world. Rome: FAO; 2020.
2. Loopstra R, Tarasuk V. The relationship between food banks and household food insecurity among low-income Toronto families. Can Public Policy. 2012;38(4):497–514.
3. Scott C, Sutherland J, Taylor A. Affordability of the UK's Eatwell guide. London: The Food Foundation; 2018.
4. Popkin BM. Nutrition transition and the global diabetes epidemic. Curr Diab Rep. 2015;15(9):64.
5. Black RE, Victoria CG, Walker SP. Maternal and child undernutrition and overweight in low-income and middle-income countries. Lancet. 2013;382(9890):427–51.

6. Rollins NC, Bhandari N, Hajeebhoy N, Horton S, Lutter CK, Martines JC, et al. Why invest, and what it will take to improve breastfeeding practices? Lancet. 2016;387(10017):491–504.

7. Victora CG, de Onis M, Hallal PC, Blössner M, Shrimpton R. Worldwide timing of growth faltering: revisiting implications for interventions. Pediatrics. 2010;125(3):e473–80.

8. Lozoff B, Beard J, Connor J, Felt B, Georgieff M, Schallert T. Long-lasting neural and behavioural effects of iron deficiency in infancy. Nutr Rev. 2006;64(5 Pt 2):S34–43.

9. Misra M, Pacaud D, Petryk A, Collett-Solberg PF, Kappy M. Vitamin D deficiency in children and its management: review of current knowledge and recommendations. Pediatrics. 2008;122(2):398–417.

10. Patton GC, Sawyer SM, Santelli JS, Ross DA, Afifi R, Allen NB, et al. Our future: a Lancet commission on adolescent health and wellbeing. Lancet. 2016;387(10036):2423–78.

11. Best JR, Miller PH. A developmental perspective on executive function. Child Dev. 2010;81(6):1641–60.

12. Lobstein T, Baur L, Uauy R. Obesity in children and young people: a crisis in public health. Obes Rev. 2004;5(s1):4–85.

13. Public Health England (PHE). Health matters: obesity and the food environment. London: PHE; 2017.

14. The Lancet. COVID-19: remaking the social contract. The Lancet. 2020 May;395(10234):1401.

15. Beatty C, Fothergill S. The local and regional impact of the UK's welfare reforms. Camb J Reg Econ Soc., 2014;7(1):63–79.

16. Marmot M, Goldblatt P, Allen J, Boyce T, McNeish D, Grady M, et al. Fair society, healthy lives (The Marmot Review). London: UCL Institute of Health Equity; 2010.

17. Forsey A. Hungry holidays: a report on hunger amongst children during school holidays. London: All-Party Parliamentary Group on Hunger; 2017.

18. The Trussell Trust. End of year stats. Salisbury: The Trussell Trust; 2019.

19. Garthwaite K. Stigma, shame and 'people like us': an ethnographic study of foodbank use in the UK. J Poverty Soc Justice. 2016;24(3):277–89.

20. Power M, Doherty B, Small N, Teasdale S, Pickett KE. All in it together? Community food aid in a multi-ethnic context. J Soc Policy. 2018;47(3):1–19.

21. Lambie-Mumford H. Hungry Britain: the rise of food charity. Bristol: Policy Press; 2017.

22. Jones NR, Conklin AI, Suhrcke M, Monsivais P. The growing price gap between more and less healthy foods: analysis of a novel longitudinal UK dataset. PLoS One. 2014;9(10):e109343.

23. Wrieden WL, Anderson AS, Longbottom PJ, Valentine K, Stead M, Caraher M, et al. The impact of a community-based food skills intervention on cooking confidence, food preparation methods and dietary choices - an exploratory trial. Public Health Nutr. 2007 Feb;10(2):203–11.

24. Joseph Rowntree Foundation (JRF). UK poverty 2019/20. York: JRF; 2020.

25. Macleod M, Curl A, Kearns A. Understanding the prevalence and drivers of food bank use: evidence from deprived communities in Glasgow. Soc Policy Soc. 2019;18(1):67–86.
26. Taras H. Nutrition and student performance at school. J Sch Health. 2005;75(6):199–213.
27. Bryan J, Osendarp S, Hughes D, Calvaresi E, Baghurst K, Van Klinken JW. Nutrients for cognitive development in school-aged children. Nutr Rev. 2004;62(8):295–306.
28. Florence MD, Asbridge M, Veugelers PJ. Diet quality and academic performance. J Sch Health. 2008;78(4):209–15.
29. Defeyter MA, Graham PL, Walton J, Apicella T. Breakfast clubs: availability for British schoolchildren and the nutritional, social and academic benefits. Nutr Bull. 2010;35(3):245–53.
30. UNICEF. The state of the world's children 2019: children, food and nutrition. New York: UNICEF; 2019.
31. Han JC, Lawlor DA, Kimm SY. Childhood obesity—2010: progress and challenges. Lancet. 2010;375(9727):1737–48.
32. Victora CG, Adair L, Fall C, Hallal PC, Martorell R, Richter L, et al. Maternal and child undernutrition: consequences for adult health and human capital. Lancet. 2008;371(9609):340–57.
33. Reilly JJ, El-Hamdouchi A, Diouf A, Monyeki A, Somda SA. Determining the worldwide prevalence of obesity. Lancet. 2018;391(10132):1773–4.
34. Gundersen C, Ziliak JP. Food insecurity and health outcomes. Health Aff. 2015;34(11):1830–9.
35. Shonkoff JP, Garner AS. The lifelong effects of early childhood adversity and toxic stress. Pediatrics. 2012;129(1):e232–46.
36. Becker CB, Middlemass K, Taylor B, Johnson C, Gomez F. Food insecurity and eating disorder pathology. Int J Eat Disord. 2017;50(9):1031–40.
37. van Lancker W, Parolin Z. COVID-19, school closures, and child poverty: a social crisis in the making. Lancet Public Health. 2020;5(5):e243–4.
38. The Trussell Trust. Lockdown, lifelines and the long haul ahead: the impact of COVID-19 on food banks in the Trussell trust network. Salisbury: The Trussell Trust; 2020.
39. O'Connell R, Knight A, Brannen J. Living hand to mouth: children and food in low-income families. Childhood. 2019;26(4):491–507.
40. Lucas PJ, Patterson E, Sacks G, Billich N, Evans CEL. Preschool and school meal policies: an overview of what we know about regulation, implementation, and impact on diet in the UK, Sweden, and Australia. Nutrients. 2017;9(7):736.
41. Rowan Hevesi, Downey M, Harvey K. Living in food insecurity: a qualitative study exploring parents' food parenting practices and their perceptions of the impact of food insecurity on their children's eating. Appetite. 2024 Jan 1;195:107204-4.
42. Hobbs JE. Food supply chains during the COVID-19 pandemic. Can J Agric Econ. 2020;68(2):171–6.
43. Power M, Doherty B, Pybus K. How COVID-19 has exposed inequalities in the UK food system: the case of UK food and poverty. Nat Food. 2020;1(6):315.

44. Pietrobelli A, Pecoraro L, Ferruzzi A, Heo M, Faith M, Zoller T, et al. Effects of COVID-19 lockdown on lifestyle behaviours in children with obesity living in Verona, Italy: a longitudinal study. Obesity (Silver Spring). 2020;28(8):1382–5.

45. Green F. Schoolwork in lockdown: new evidence on the epidemic of educational poverty. London: Centre for Learning and Life Chances in Knowledge Economies and Societies (LLAKES); 2020.

46. Andrew A, Cattan S, Costa Dias M, Farquharson C, Kraftman L, Krutikova S, et al. Inequalities in children's experiences of home learning during the COVID-19 lockdown in England. Fiscal Stud. 2020;41(3):653–83.

47. Office of the Children's Commissioner. Tackling the disadvantage gap during the COVID-19 crisis. London: Children's Commissioner; 2020.

48. Galobardes B, Lynch JW, Smith GD. Childhood socioeconomic circumstances and cause-specific mortality in adulthood: systematic review and interpretation. Epidemiol Rev. 2004;26:7–21.

49. Barker DJP. The developmental origins of adult disease. J Am Coll Nutr. 2004;23(sup6):588S–95S.

50. Forrester T, Barker D, Fall C. Fetal programming and obesity. Springer; 2018.

51. Smith LC, Meade B. Measuring food insecurity in crisis situations: evidence from Ethiopia and Darfur. Food Policy. 2019;86:101725.

52. Wadsworth ME, Raviv T, Santiago CD, Etter EM. Testing the adaptation to poverty-related stress model: predicting low-income children's coping and psychological adjustment. J Clin Child Adolesc Psychol. 2011;40(4):646–57.

53. Scarborough P, Bhatnagar P, Wickramasinghe KK, Allender S, Foster C, Rayner M. The economic burden of ill health due to diet, physical inactivity, smoking, alcohol and obesity in the UK: an update to 2006–07 NHS costs. J Public Health (Oxf). 2011;33(4):527–35.

54. World Health Organization (WHO). A conceptual framework for action on the social determinants of health. Geneva: WHO; 2010.

55. Department for Education. Free school meals guidance. London: Department for Education; 2018.

56. The Children's Society. Free school meals and poverty. London: The Children's Society; 2019.

57. Ministry of Housing, Communities & Local Government (MHCLG). Homelessness reduction act 2017: policy factsheets. London: MHCLG; 2018.

58. HM Government. Chancellor of the exchequer's statement on coronavirus (COVID-19). London: HM Government; 2020.

59. Parnham, JC, Chang, K, Rauber, F, Levy RB, Laverty AA, Pearson-Stuttard, J, et al. Evaluating the impact of the universal infant free school meal policy on the ultra-processed food content of children's lunches in England and Scotland: a natural experiment. Int J Behav Nutr Phys Act. 2024;21:124.

60. Morgan K, Sonnino R. The school food revolution: public food and the challenge of sustainable development. London: Earthscan; 2010.

61. Dimbleby H. National food strategy: part one. London: HM Government; 2020.
62. Condliffe S, Link CR. The relationship between economic status and child health: evidence from the United States. Am Econ Rev. 2008;98(4):1605–18.
63. Public Health England (PHE). Sugar reduction: the evidence for action. London: PHE; 2015.
64. Marmot M, Allen J, Goldblatt P, Herd E, Morrison J. Build back fairer: the COVID-19 marmot review. London: Institute of Health Equity; 2020.
65. Sosenko F, Bramley G, Bhattacharjee A. Understanding the post-2010 increase in food bank use in England: new quasi-experimental analysis of the role of welfare policy. BMC Public Health [Internet]. 2022 Jul 16;22(1). Available from: https://bmcpublichealth.biomedcentral.com/articles/10.1186/s12889-022-13738-0
66. Loopstra R. Vulnerability to food insecurity since the COVID-19 lockdown. London: Food Foundation; 2020.
67. Zorbas C, Browne J, Chung A, Peeters A, Booth S, Pollard C, et al. Shifting the social determinants of food insecurity during the COVID-19 pandemic: the Australian experience. Food Security. 2022 Sep 17.
68. Purdam K, Garratt EA, Esmail A. Hungry? Food insecurity, social stigma and embarrassment in the UK. Sociology. 2016;50(6):1072–88.
69. Bartfeld JS, Ahn HM. The school breakfast program strengthens household food security among low-income households with elementary school children. J Nutr. 2011;141(3):470–5.
70. Dowler E. Food banks and food justice in 'Austerity Britain'. In: Riches G, Silvasti T, editors. First world hunger revisited. London: Palgrave Macmillan; 2014. p. 160–75.
71. Taylor A, Loopstra R. Too poor to eat: food insecurity in the UK. London: Food Foundation; 2016.
72. BBC News. Marcus Rashford: campaigning footballer calls for policy change on child hunger. 2020 Jun 16.
73. House of Commons Library. School meals and nutritional standards (England). London: House of Commons; 2021.

3 Homelessness

3.1 Historical Overview: Housing Inequality Prior to COVID-19

3.1.1 From Post-War Reconstruction to Austerity

British housing policy has gone through numerous transformations since the post-Second World War era. The massive construction of council housing in the mid-20th century attempted to address acute shortages and poor-quality housing stock. Yet, as the decades wore on, policies such as the right to buy scheme—introduced in 1980 under the Housing Act—triggered a major shift in tenure patterns, drastically diminishing the pool of social housing available to those on lower incomes (1). Concurrently, insufficient reinvestment in new social housing stock led to a structural imbalance in housing supply and demand. By the 1990s, it was evident that rising private rents, deregulation, and the undermining of local authorities' ability to build social housing would culminate in significant long-term pressure on the housing system (2).

Austerity policies from 2010 onwards further curtailed local authority budgets and welfare spending, exacerbating the existing crisis. In particular, cuts to housing benefits—coupled with a dearth of affordable housing, especially in high-cost urban areas—created conditions where precarious living situations became the norm for low-income households (3). The cost burden of private rents and unstable work patterns left many households teetering on the brink of homelessness. These trends played a direct role in the fragmentation of communities, as families that once could afford to live in certain areas became displaced, leading to severed social networks and educational disruptions for children (4).

3.1.2 Housing Tenure and Health Inequalities

Housing tenure, whether one owns, rents privately, or rents socially, is closely tied to both economic security and physical and mental health outcomes. Research consistently demonstrates that individuals in lower-quality private rental housing are more likely to experience stress, respiratory illnesses (due

DOI: 10.4324/9781003312529-4

to damp and mould), and a higher risk of accidental injuries (5). Statutory homelessness, a status that local authorities grant when individuals or families meet specific criteria for being homeless or at risk of homelessness, represents just the tip of the iceberg. Hidden homelessness—people "sofa-surfing" or living in unregulated temporary arrangements—complicates attempts to gauge the full scale of housing insecurity (6).

Socioeconomic disparities overlap with health inequalities in a vicious cycle: households struggling with unemployment, low pay, or chronic illnesses often lack the capital to secure better housing, which in turn perpetuates poor health outcomes. The high cost of housing in regions such as London and the South East tends to funnel lower-income households into deprived neighbourhoods where schools, healthcare facilities, and employment opportunities are also under strain (7). These layers of disadvantage cultivate powerful feedback loops, locking vulnerable populations into precarious living conditions, financial instability, and compromised health.

3.1.3   Inadequate Policy Responses Before the Pandemic

Before COVID-19, government-led interventions to tackle homelessness and housing insecurity were often short-term, failing to address structural causes. The Homelessness Reduction Act 2017 aimed to place additional duties on councils to prevent homelessness, but in practice local authorities found themselves overwhelmed by limited funding and the sheer volume of households seeking assistance (8). Efforts to reduce rough sleeping—such as the rough sleeping initiative—produced some positive outcomes at local levels, yet did not reverse the national upward trend (9). Furthermore, many local authorities faced bureaucratic hurdles, including rigid eligibility criteria for statutory homelessness, leaving numerous single adults, and those with no recourse to public funds unsupported.

In the lead-up to the pandemic, numerous think tanks and academic researchers warned of an impending housing "tipping point", wherein further economic shocks could send tens of thousands more households into homelessness. Their forecasts proved accurate: as the pandemic struck, entire swaths of the population were pushed closer to the brink due to sudden unemployment, reduced household incomes, and mounting rental arrears (10). Without a robust safety net or sufficient temporary accommodation stock, the resultant surge in housing need laid bare the stark fragility of Britain's housing ecosystem.

3.2   Magnitude and Manifestations of Homelessness in Pre-Pandemic Britain

3.2.1   Defining Homelessness in the British Context

Homelessness in Britain is a multifaceted phenomenon. The official statutory definition pertains to those who lack a safe, legal residence and qualify for assistance from local authorities. However, many individuals who do not meet the strict criteria of "priority need" remain categorised as "non-statutory homeless" and often fall through the cracks, receiving minimal or no support (11). This category encompasses hidden homelessness, such as overcrowded or informal living arrangements, where people rely on friends and family for shelter without the stability of a tenancy agreement. Rough sleeping, although perhaps the most visible manifestation of homelessness, represents only a fraction of those experiencing housing insecurity (12).

3.2.2   National Trends and Key Demographics

Government statistics revealed a gradual but concerning rise in the number of statutory homeless households in the years preceding COVID-19 (8, 10). Local authority records consistently showed that families, single parents (particularly mothers), and young people were among the fastest-growing groups in need. Concurrently, rough sleeping figures also escalated, with the department for levelling up, housing, and communities reporting a marked increase from 2010 onwards (13). Women sleeping rough, although less visible, were reported to be at higher risk of violence and exploitation, demonstrating the need for gender-specific interventions (14).

People from ethnic minority backgrounds have faced disproportionate risks of homelessness, with structural racism compounding financial disadvantage and limiting access to suitable housing (15). Migrants with no recourse to public funds were often excluded from statutory homelessness support, intensifying their vulnerability. Additionally, the research highlighted the higher incidence of homelessness among individuals who had experienced trauma, mental health conditions, or disruptions in social support networks such as care leavers (16).

3.2.3   Health Burden and Social Costs

The health implications of homelessness—even pre-pandemic—are stark. Homeless individuals experience far higher rates of morbidity and mortality compared to their housed counterparts, with infections, respiratory illnesses, mental health disorders, and substance dependency being common (17). Chronic stress associated with insecure housing intensifies the likelihood of non-communicable diseases such as hypertension and diabetes (18). Furthermore, homelessness often contributes to precarious employment, creating a cycle of poverty that is extremely difficult to break.

Public costs accrue in various ways, from increased demands on the NHS and social services to greater involvement with the criminal justice system. Evidence suggests that targeted supportive housing can reduce these costs significantly, but consistent investment in such interventions was lacking prior to

COVID-19 (19). These findings underscore the interrelated nature of housing, health, and social well-being—neglecting one domain triggers negative ripple effects across the others.

3.3 Policy Measures and Their (In)Effectiveness Before COVID-19

3.3.1 The Homelessness Reduction Act: A Partial Solution

Enacted to expand local authorities' duties to prevent and relieve homelessness, the Homelessness Reduction Act 2017 marked a noteworthy legislative shift. It mandated councils to intervene at earlier stages and offer more personalised plans (8). Yet critics argued that the Act's potential was undermined by insufficient funding and the overarching constraints of austerity (20). Many authorities simply did not have the capacity or resources to cope with the increased demand, leaving numerous vulnerable individuals and families in limbo. Moreover, the Act's focus on prevention and relief often relied on the availability of affordable housing options, which in many areas remained elusive.

3.3.2 Limitations in Social Housing Provision

Social housing is frequently hailed as one of the most effective levers for mitigating homelessness, yet the reality in Britain has been one of persistent shortfall. Policies that sold off council properties without replacing them at scale eroded the social housing stock, particularly in high-demand urban regions (1). Successive governments introduced schemes encouraging homeownership—such as Help to Buy—thereby shifting policy focus away from building truly affordable rental units.

The interplay between private markets and social housing remains critical. As private rents continue to soar in many parts of Britain, low-income households depend on local authorities to provide social housing or subsidise rents through housing benefits. But where social housing remains constrained, people end up in temporary accommodations, often for prolonged periods. Temporary accommodation placements soared before COVID-19, signifying a failure in upstream solutions (21).

3.3.3 The Unresolved Challenge of "No Recourse to Public Funds"

A subgroup particularly hard hit by housing insecurity comprises migrants who fall under the "no recourse to public funds" (NRPF) condition. This legal restriction denies them access to mainstream welfare benefits, including most housing support schemes (22). Prior to COVID-19, this group's living conditions were frequently precarious, relying on informal networks or exploitative living arrangements. The statutory system was largely not prepared to manage the complex and urgent needs of individuals with NRPF, pushing many into destitution. The broader implications—such as undocumented migrants avoiding healthcare for fear of enforcement—further complicated public health measures, underscoring how housing insecurity can intersect with wider issues of social marginalisation.

3.4 COVID-19 and the Worsening of Housing Insecurity

3.4.1 The Early Pandemic Response

When COVID-19 struck, the importance of "staying at home" as the primary defence against viral transmission underscored the inequality faced by those without a home. In March 2020, the UK Government launched the "Everyone In" initiative—a policy instructing local authorities to provide emergency accommodation for rough sleepers to protect them from the virus (23). This measure was initially lauded for its rapid mobilisation, which saw thousands of people moved into hotels and other temporary settings almost overnight.

Despite its successes, "Everyone In" was not a permanent solution. Critics observed that the scheme's eligibility criteria evolved over time, leaving some vulnerable groups excluded (24). Additionally, local authorities experienced difficulties in transitioning individuals out of these hotels into long-term suitable housing. While "Everyone In" demonstrated that a robust, well-funded strategy could markedly reduce rough sleeping, its short-term nature left many questioning whether it was merely a temporary fix rather than a paradigm shift in tackling homelessness.

3.4.2 Economic Shock, Evictions, and Arrears

COVID-19 delivered a significant economic blow, with widespread job losses in sectors such as hospitality, retail, and the arts. Households experiencing unemployment or reduced working hours struggled to keep up with rent or mortgage payments (25). Though measures like the furlough scheme and temporary increases in Universal Credit helped some households to stay afloat, others accrued substantial rental arrears. Furthermore, the temporary eviction ban introduced during the height of the pandemic did not necessarily halt the accrual of debt, effectively deferring a potential avalanche of evictions once the moratorium ended (26).

For private renters—who are disproportionately younger, lower-income, and without assets to fall back on—the end of the eviction ban led to a surge in notices to quit. Indeed, research by homelessness charities and academic institutions indicated a sharp rise in households seeking council support due to rent arrears post-lockdown (27). Consequently, Britain faced a new wave of statutory homelessness applications, revealing the precarious state of housing security for millions, even those who had never before engaged with council housing services.

3.4.3 Health Implications During the Pandemic

In overcrowded or substandard housing, the basic public health guidance of "self-isolation" or "social distancing" became nearly impossible. Overcrowded households encountered higher rates of transmission, particularly among multi-generational families (28). Additionally, those who were already homeless or living in emergency accommodations often lacked consistent access to sanitation facilities, making public health measures such as frequent hand-washing challenging to maintain (17). The stress of pandemic-related uncertainty, coupled with cramped living conditions, escalated mental health concerns, as highlighted in various Public Health England briefings (29).

Notably, the link between housing and underlying health conditions was further amplified by COVID-19. People in poor-quality, damp, or cold homes were more prone to respiratory issues, potentially increasing vulnerability to the virus (5). Meanwhile, individuals with multiple comorbidities who were also homeless or inadequately housed faced compound risks of severe illness and mortality (30). The pandemic effectively shone a harsh spotlight on the health burden of housing inequality, which had been festering for decades.

3.5 The Case of Statutory Homelessness

3.5.1 Growing Statutory Homelessness During COVID-19

Though exact figures vary, local authorities reported a substantial increase in statutory homelessness applications through 2020–2021 (31). This upturn was partly driven by tenants who fell behind on rent due to lost income, and partly by individuals exiting precarious informal arrangements. Domestic abuse survivors, who had fewer escape routes during lockdowns, also presented in growing numbers, underscoring the interplay between public health measures and personal safety (32). The capacity of local authorities to respond was further constrained by staff shortages, remote working, and the broader strains on public services.

3.5.2 Administrative Barriers and Eligibility Criteria

Eligibility for statutory homelessness support remains rooted in complex legal criteria regarding priority need, intentionality, and local connection (33). These stipulations disqualify many people from assistance, including single adults without dependents or individuals who cannot evidence a local link. Such barriers were particularly problematic during the pandemic, as people who could not demonstrate a stable residence history found themselves excluded from emergency housing allocations, despite facing acute homelessness risks. The reduced scope of housing benefits and local housing allowance rates in high-rent areas further impeded the ability of councils to find suitable placements.

3.5.3   The "Quick Fix" of Temporary Accommodation

Local authorities increasingly resorted to placing homeless households in temporary accommodation—bed-and-breakfasts, hostels, or even disused office blocks—particularly as the pandemic surged (8). While preferable to rough sleeping, these setups often lack privacy, sanitation facilities, or the wrap-around services needed to address complex needs such as mental illness or addiction (19). Prolonged stays in temporary accommodation also undermine family stability, particularly for children who may find it challenging to maintain consistent schooling and social networks. As these placements became prolonged during the pandemic, the risk of institutionalising housing insecurity and normalising substandard conditions grew.

3.6   Societal Consequences of Inadequate Housing During the Pandemic

3.6.1   Educational Disruptions

One of the most profound societal repercussions of Britain's housing instability has been the disruption to children's education, a phenomenon that escalated during COVID-19. Families living in temporary accommodation or overcrowded conditions had limited capacity to support remote learning. Lacking stable internet access, quiet study spaces, or consistent routines, children experienced academic regression and deteriorating mental well-being (34). The closure of libraries, youth clubs, and community centres removed additional educational and social buffers. While educational disruption affected students across the socioeconomic spectrum, those already contending with homelessness or housing insecurity suffered disproportionately, exacerbating educational inequalities (35).

3.6.2   Labour Market Vulnerability

The pandemic inflicted a major shock on Britain's labour market. As unemployment rose, competition for jobs intensified, placing those with unstable housing at a distinct disadvantage. Individuals without a permanent address often struggled to apply for jobs or verify their residence for administrative processes (25). The cyclical interplay of precarious work and housing insecurity became more apparent: living in insecure housing can hamper employability, while job loss or reduced hours can easily precipitate arrears and eviction. The broader outcome is a cluster of socioeconomic disadvantages that can reverberate through entire lifetimes.

3.6.3 Mental Health Costs

Housing instability exerts a profound impact on psychological well-being, an effect aggravated by the isolation and uncertainty of COVID-19. Many individuals in precarious living conditions reported heightened anxiety and depression, driven by fears of infection, economic hardship, and potential eviction (29). Children in such environments showed elevated indicators of distress, including difficulties in emotional regulation, often requiring additional support from already overstretched social services (36). Even after restrictions were lifted, the mental health legacies of pandemic-related housing insecurity persisted, with some experts referring to an "echo pandemic" of mental health disorders (37).

3.6.4 Social Cohesion and Community Resilience

Finally, the erosion of safe, stable housing undermines social cohesion. Communities reliant on high turnover private rentals often struggle to foster robust neighbourhood networks, rendering them less able to support each other during crises. Social capital—embodied by community centres, food banks, and local initiatives—can be stunted by constant population flux. The pandemic tested Britain's capacity for community-based resilience: while some neighbourhoods rallied around mutual aid groups, others were hampered by the transience caused by evictions or lack of public services (38). Thus, housing stability stands as a cornerstone of social resilience, enabling communities to collectively respond to emergencies and support their most vulnerable members.

3.7 Post-Pandemic Ramifications: The Lost Generation of COVID-19

3.7.1 Long-Term Health Inequalities

As the immediate crisis of COVID-19 recedes, Britain faces a landscape marred by deepened health inequalities. Delayed medical care, neglected chronic conditions, and increased mental health strain will exacerbate pre-existing gaps between socioeconomically advantaged and disadvantaged groups (39). Homeless individuals and families, who already suffer disproportionately from untreated conditions, may bear the brunt of these delayed health consequences. The risk of a "lost generation" of children and young adults, whose physical and mental health was compromised during this period, looms large.

3.7.2   Intergenerational Consequences

Housing insecurity will likely reverberate across generations, affecting everything from educational attainment to labour market performance. Young people who watched their families struggle to maintain stable housing during the pandemic may find themselves less optimistic about future prospects, with dampened ambitions and persistent emotional scars. In the academic literature, adverse childhood experiences are firmly associated with poorer health outcomes and reduced socioeconomic achievements later in life (40). Given the scale of housing insecurity during COVID-19, concerns grow around a cohort shaped by recurring displacement, financial precariousness, and relentless anxiety.

3.7.3   The Risk of Normalising Temporary Solutions

A critical question emerges: might the extraordinary measures taken during the pandemic—like hotel placements and eviction bans—devolve into a patchwork approach rather than spurring systematic reform? Evidence from previous crises suggests that short-term relief can indeed catalyse more sustained policy transformations, but this is by no means guaranteed (9). If the momentum for change fizzles, Britain risks settling into a new normal where makeshift accommodations, precarious private tenancies, and repeated disruptions are seen as unavoidable realities of the housing landscape. This outcome would entrench existing inequalities and perpetuate cycles of homelessness well into the future.

3.8   Future Directions and Concluding Remarks

3.8.1   Pathways for Policy Transformation

The pandemic has made it abundantly clear that decent housing is essential for public health, social stability, and personal dignity. If there is a silver lining to be found, it lies in the collective realisation of housing's foundational role in societal well-being. A coherent post-pandemic strategy could include:

1. Scaling Up Social Housing: A renewed commitment to expanding social housing supply, particularly in high-demand areas, could alleviate pressure

on private rental markets and provide stable, long-term homes for vulnerable households (1). This would require ring-fenced funding for local authorities and a revision of restrictive planning regulations.

2. Overhauling Statutory Homelessness Criteria: Streamlining eligibility requirements to ensure that the hidden homeless populations, single adults, and those with NRPF are not perpetually excluded from vital housing support (22). Local authorities must be backed with resources that enable more holistic and long-term solutions, including wrap-around healthcare and social services.

3. Rent Controls and Tenant Protections: Given the volatility and high cost of private renting, measures such as rent caps, longer-term tenancies, and strengthened eviction protections could offer some security to tenants (41). These initiatives must be balanced to ensure viability for landlords but with the core aim of preventing avoidable evictions and housing instability.

4. Integration of Health and Housing Services: By closely aligning housing policy with public health objectives, Britain can better address the underlying social determinants of health (42). Joint commissioning of housing and health services, funded by devolved budgets, may offer a more nuanced, localised approach that tackles root causes rather than patching up symptoms.

3.8.2   Opportunities for Grassroots and Community-Led Solutions

While top-down policy reforms are essential, grassroots interventions can play a pivotal role in mitigating housing inequalities. Community land trusts, cooperative housing models, and local activism offer ways to empower residents, manage rents, and secure tenure. Such initiatives can bolster local resilience, foster social cohesion, and enable marginalised voices to shape housing developments (43). The pandemic, paradoxically, ignited new forms of community solidarity—via food banks, mutual aid groups, and informal support networks. Harnessing this collective spirit can help amplify grassroots responses that push for radical housing solutions.

3.8.3   A Closing Call to Action

Housing has emerged from the pandemic not merely as a commodity but as a public health imperative and moral touchstone. The stark lesson gleaned from COVID-19 is that substandard, insecure, or unaffordable housing compromises every aspect of life—from physical health to educational prospects, mental well-being, and social mobility. As Britain strives to rebuild a fairer, more resilient society, the question is whether we will seize the impetus to invest in comprehensive housing reform or resort to a patchwork of short-lived measures.

Addressing housing inequalities goes beyond politics; it is a critical step in safeguarding public health, enhancing social stability, and restoring trust in institutions. For the countless individuals and families who have experienced homelessness or live one paycheque away from eviction, the stakes are immeasurable. Beyond the moral imperative lies a pragmatic consideration: no society can thrive when large segments of its population are consigned to the margins. We have the evidence, the tools, and the impetus—now we must summon the collective will to transform insight into lasting change.

References

1. Murie A. Right to buy: history and prospect. Hous Stud. 2016;31(3):303–17.
2. Bambra C, Barr A, Brown B, Davies H, Konstantinos H, Mason D, et al. Tackling inequalities for UK health and productivity; 2020.
3. Hudson-Sharp N, Munro-Lott N, Rolfe H, Runge J. The impact of welfare reform and welfare-to- work programmes: an evidence review. Equality and Human Rights Commission Research Report; 2018.
4. Savage M. Revealed: homeless children spending entire lives in temporary housing in England. The Observer. 2024 Mar 9.
5. Liddell C, Guiney C. Living in a cold and damp home: frameworks for understanding impacts on mental well-being. Public Health. 2015;129(3):191–9.
6. Bramley G, Fitzpatrick S, Wood J, Sosenko F, Blenkinsopp J. State of the nation: understanding homelessness in the UK. Institute for Social Policy, Housing and Equalities Research; 2019. Report No.: 46.
7. Office for National Statistics (ONS). Socioeconomic inequalities in housing across England. London: ONS; 2020.
8. Ministry of Housing, Communities & Local Government (MHCLG). Homelessness reduction act 2017: policy factsheets. London: MHCLG; 2018.
9. Fitzpatrick S, Pawson H, Bramley G, Wilcox S, Watts B. The homelessness monitor: England 2020. London: Crisis; 2020.
10. Clarke A, Hamilton C, Jones M, Muir K. Poverty, evictions and forced moves. Joseph Rowntree Foundation; 2017. Report No.: 117.
11. Mackie P. Varieties of homelessness governance: a comparative analysis in Europe. Int J Hous Policy. 2019;19(1):1–5.
12. Aldridge RW, Story A, Hwang SW, Noori T, Luchenski SA, Hayward AC, et al. Morbidity and mortality in homeless individuals, prisoners, sex workers, and individuals with substance use disorders in high-income countries: a systematic review and meta-analysis. Lancet. 2018;391(10117):241–50.
13. Department for Levelling Up, Housing & Communities (DLUHC). Rough sleeping snapshot in England: Autumn 2019. London: DLUHC; 2020.
14. Bretherton J, Pleace N. Women and rough sleeping: a critical review of current research and methodology. University of York, Centre for Housing Policy; 2018. Report No.: 08.

15. Netto G. Strangers in the city: addressing challenges to the protection, housing and settlement of refugees. Int J Hous Policy. 2011;11(3):285–303.
16. Self T, Miles H, Harding B. The relationships between youth homelessness and offending: A systematic review of the UK literature. Children and Youth Serv Rev. 2024 Nov 22;108032.
17. Story A. Slopes and cliffs in health inequalities: comparative morbidity of housed and homeless people. Lancet. 2013;382(S3):S93.
18. Fazel S, Geddes JR, Kushel M. The health of homeless people in high-income countries: descriptive epidemiology, health consequences, and clinical and policy recommendations. Lancet. 2014;384(9953):1529–40.
19. Housing First England. Evaluation of housing first services in England. Homeless Link; 2019. Report No.: HF1.
20. Beatty C, Fothergill S. Welfare reform in the UK 2010–16: expectations, outcomes, and local impacts. Soc Policy Admin. 2018;52(5):659–78.
21. Shelter. Denied the right to a safe home: temporary accommodation. London: Shelter; 2019.
22. Price J, Spencer S, Pierce M. Migrants with no recourse to public funds: the implications for local authorities. COMPAS; 2020. Report No.: 14.
23. Ministry of Housing, Communities & Local Government (MHCLG). Coronavirus (COVID-19) emergency accommodation survey data: May 2020. London: MHCLG; 2020.
24. The Kerslake Commission on Homelessness and Rough Sleeping. A new way of working: ending rough sleeping together. The Kerslake Commission; 2021. Interim Report.
25. Blundell R, Costa Dias M, Joyce R, Xu X. COVID-19 and inequalities. Fisc Stud. 2020;41(2):291–319.
26. MHCLG. Understanding the possession action process: guidance for landlords and tenants. London: MHCLG; 2021.
27. Versey HS. The impending eviction cliff: Housing insecurity during COVID-19. Am J Public Health. 2021 Aug;111(8):1423–7.
28. Ghosh AK, Venkatraman S, Soroka O, Reshetnyak E, Rajan M, An A, et al. Association between overcrowded households, multigenerational households, and COVID-19: a cohort study. Public Health. 2021 Sep;198:273–9.
29. Public Health England. COVID-19 mental health and wellbeing surveillance report. London: PHE; 2021.
30. Lewer D, Aldridge RW, Menezes D, Sawyer C, Zaninotto P, Dedicoat M, et al. Health-related quality of life and prevalence of six chronic diseases in homeless and housed people: a cross-sectional study in London and Birmingham, England. Arch Public Health. 2021;79:33.
31. Department for Levelling Up, Housing & Communities (DLUHC). Statutory homelessness in England: 2020–2021. London: DLUHC; 2021.
32. Women's Aid. A perfect storm: the impact of the COVID-19 pandemic on domestic abuse survivors and the services supporting them. Women's Aid; 2020.
33. MHCLG. Homelessness code of guidance for local authorities. London: MHCLG; 2018.

34. Andrew A, Cattan S, Costa Dias M, Farquharson C, Kraftman L, Krutik-ova S, et al. Inequalities in children's experiences of home learning during the COVID-19 lockdown in England. Fisc Stud. 2020;41(3):653–83.
35. Cullinane C, Montacute R. COVID-19 and social mobility impact brief #1: school shutdown. Sutton Trust; 2020. Report No.: ST001.
36. Mental Health Foundation. Impacts of lockdown on mental health. London: MHF; 2021.
37. Pierce M, Hope H, Abel KM, Hatch S, Hotopf M, John A, et al. Mental health before and during the COVID-19 pandemic: a longitudinal probability sample survey of the UK population. Lancet Psychiatry. 2020;7(10):883–92.
38. Butler P. Covid has exposed dire position of England's local councils. the Guardian. The Guardian; 2021 Jul 10.
39. Marmot M, Allen J, Goldblatt P, Herd E, Morrison J. Build back fairer: the COVID-19 marmot review. London: Institute of Health Equity; 2020.
40. Bellis MA, Hughes K, Leckenby N, Perkins C, Lowey H. National household survey of adverse childhood experiences and their relationship with resilience to health-harming behaviours in England. BMC Med. 2014;12:72.
41. Whitehead C, Williams P. Assessing the evidence on rent control from an international perspective. London: LSE; 2018.
42. World Health Organization (WHO). Housing and health guidelines. Geneva: WHO; 2018.
43. Moore T, McKee K. Empowering local communities? An international review of community land trusts. Hous Stud. 2012;27(2):280–90.

4   Mental Health

Introduction

The Lost Generation of COVID-19: A Critical Analysis of Health and Social Inequality in Post-Pandemic Britain demands that we confront a profound yet often invisible crisis: the mental health catastrophe that has engulfed our youngest citizens. While the world has tracked hospital admissions and economic shocks, the more insidious damage—the emotional turmoil of children—is only just coming into focus. Surging anxiety, stunted social development, and heartbreaking loneliness have coalesced into a mental health epidemic that is likely to outlast the virus itself.

Even before COVID-19, Britain's mental health system was underfunded and unprepared, leaving many children languishing on waiting lists or without any support at all (1). The pandemic pried open these long-standing cracks, slamming vulnerable children with abrupt school closures, digital isolation, family stress, and economic strain. Far too many now face a precarious future, their once manageable difficulties—whether mild anxiety or early signs of depression—amplified into a severe mental health crisis. For those in disadvantaged communities, the stakes are even higher: pandemic hardships have deepened the gulf between children with resources and those without. This chapter unpacks how the pandemic unleashed a silent epidemic of distress among Britain's children, threatening to create a "lost generation" shaped by chronic mental health inequalities.

4.1   Fragile Foundations: Pre-Pandemic Inequalities in Child Mental Health

4.1.1   Existing Fault Lines

Children's mental health in Britain has been on the edge of a precipice for years. Even in 2019, demand for child and adolescent mental health services far outstripped supply (2). These shortfalls collided with social determinants—poverty, racism, housing insecurity—that systematically expose certain children to chronic stress and undermine emotional

DOI: 10.4324/9781003312529-5

well-being (3). As austerity measures ravaged local authority budgets, school counsellors and community services vanished, leaving a skeletal infrastructure for youth mental health support. When COVID-19 struck, it slammed into this incomplete safety net and tore it apart.

4.1.2 Who Was Already at Risk?

The children least equipped to weather the pandemic's storm were those already living on the margins. Youth from low-income backgrounds, ethnic minorities, families experiencing homelessness, or those with SEND faced structural disadvantages in both education and health (4). Mental health problems in these groups were already rising faster than in the general population, reflecting the everyday barriers they navigated—barriers that tripled in size once lockdowns started and social support eroded.

4.2 Lockdowns and School Closures: Catalysts for Crisis

4.2.1 The Emotional Fallout of Sudden Isolation

Lockdowns severed children from their peers, teachers, and extended family in one fell swoop. For those from unstable homes—crowded flats, stressed-out households, or families grappling with job loss—the school had often been a sanctuary offering routine, social connectedness, and sometimes even regular meals (5). When that sanctuary disappeared, daily life spiralled into unpredictability. Children reported feeling trapped, lonely, and anxious, with no clear sense of when "normal" would return (6).

4.2.2 Learning Loss and Digital Divides

While remote learning rescued some semblance of education for better-resourced students, the digital chasm brutalised poorer children. Broken laptops, no broadband, cramped living spaces: these factors conspired to cut off many from lessons and peer interaction (7). Academic setbacks soon bled into emotional despair, especially for students who felt they were slipping irreversibly behind. For children whose parents could not afford tutors or, in many cases, even consistent Wi-Fi, hopelessness set in. The mental anguish of being left out—of both education and social life—was sharp.

4.2.3 The Rise in Family Stress and Abuse

As unemployment soared and household finances collapsed, home environments often became hotbeds of anxiety and tension (8). Domestic violence charities and children's helplines reported an upsurge in calls from children living in fear under lockdown. Schools that might have flagged neglect or abuse were closed. Social workers operated at a limited capacity. Children trapped in these homes had nowhere to run, locked down with abusers behind closed doors. The psychological toll is immeasurable, creating layers of trauma that can echo through a child's lifetime.

4.3 Unequal Burdens: Vulnerable Children Pushed to the Edge

4.3.1 Ethnic Minority Youth: The Double Jeopardy

For many ethnic minority children, pre-pandemic life already included discrimination, higher poverty rates, and inequalities in school funding (9). COVID-19 infections and deaths were disproportionately higher in minority communities, amplifying loss, grief, and fear. Racist scapegoating—especially towards Asian communities—further fuelled anxiety and isolation (10). These children experienced "double jeopardy", enduring both the universal strain of the pandemic and the weight of structural racism that had existed all along.

4.3.2 SEND Children: Abandoned by a Broken System

Children with SEND rely on consistent routines, therapists, classroom assistants, and specialised environments to thrive (11). Abrupt school closures and the shortage of skilled support staff left them flailing academically, socially, and emotionally. Parents described regressive behaviours, anxiety outbursts, and a desperate struggle to maintain therapy at home without professional guidance. Already precarious services were stretched thinner, leaving families to cope in isolation—a breeding ground for mental health crises.

4.3.3 Young Carers: Childhood Sacrificed

Before the pandemic, thousands of children in Britain were already functioning as young carers for ill or disabled family members (12). Lockdowns piled on extra responsibilities: with external care paused, young carers had to manage medication, personal care, and household tasks with minimal respite. Online learning became a distant dream. Mental exhaustion rose to crushing levels. Many reported feeling forgotten by a system that rarely acknowledged their hidden workload or the immense psychological weight it inflicted.

4.4 The Emotional Toll on Adolescents: Identity Lost in Quarantine

4.4.1 Social Media Frenzies and Isolation

Teenagers, wired for social experiences, found themselves exiled to bedrooms. Even though they had social media, hours of scrolling only magnified insecurities and gloom. Cyberbullying and unrelenting pandemic headlines fuelled anxiety. For LGBTQ+ adolescents in unsupportive households, the school had offered a reprieve—a place to be themselves. Now, forced closeness with disapproving relatives caused mental health to plummet (13). The conflict between needing peer connection and being confined was raw and relentless.

4.4.2 Spikes in Depression and Self-Harm

Multiple surveys indicated a surge in self-harm and suicidal ideation among teenagers, especially those contending with grief, academic meltdown, or household conflict (14). Feeling powerless and unmotivated, many withdrew into digital spaces where negative voices—internal or external—echoed louder. Accessing mental health care was challenging: face-to-face therapy sessions were cancelled, and helplines were strained under overwhelming demand. This perfect storm of emotional vulnerability and service unavailability birthed a mental health disaster.

4.5 Long COVID for the Mind: Enduring Consequences

4.5.1 Chronic Mental Health Conditions in the Making

Children's developing brains are uniquely susceptible to trauma. Prolonged stress can rewire emotional regulation, increasing the lifetime risk of anxiety, depression, and substance misuse (15). Lost months—or years—of normal schooling and social engagement may translate into entrenched psychological scars. The risk is stark: a generation of children emerging from the pandemic with chronic mental health conditions, deepening Britain's existing disparities for decades.

4.5.2 Educational and Socioeconomic Fallout

Gaps in education translate directly into long-term social and economic inequities. Children who drop behind academically during lockdown often face a heightened risk of dropping out altogether, limiting employment options and future earning potential (16). For disadvantaged children, the mental health repercussions of repeated academic failure can solidify a cycle of poverty, poor health, and reduced aspirations. This is how a mental health crisis transforms into a societal crisis, with ramifications for the very fabric of post-pandemic Britain.

4.5.3 Community Fractures

When mental health deteriorates at scale, the impact ripples through families, schools, and neighbourhoods. The resulting tensions—family breakdowns, youth violence, or substance abuse—can fracture community cohesion. Youth clubs, after-school programmes, and community spaces could help mitigate this damage, but only if significantly reinvested in. Without these lifelines, the ongoing mental health epidemic will deepen social divisions and entrench a grim legacy of disadvantage for children in the most neglected areas.

4.6 Searching for Solutions: Repairing the Damage

4.6.1 Putting Mental Health at the Centre of Child Recovery Plans

Policymakers must recognise that any post-pandemic strategy focusing on academic "catch-up" without addressing mental health is doomed to fail. Both the Treasury and local authorities should ring-fence funding for child and adolescent mental health services, ensuring that schools, social services, and community organisations can refer children quickly (17). An integrated approach—mental health professionals embedded in every school, rigorous staff training, and consistent follow-up—will be indispensable for reversing the tide.

4.6.2 Community-Based Interventions and Grassroots Approaches

Local charities, youth centres, and voluntary groups became unsung heroes during the pandemic, delivering food parcels, laptops, and emotional support. These grassroots models, rooted in trust and understanding of local needs, could form the backbone of Britain's mental health recovery (18). Funding them is crucial—not as a stopgap measure but as a cornerstone of rebuilding. Initiatives like peer-support networks, art and sports therapy, and culturally informed counselling can help children reconnect with others and process their trauma in a safe environment.

4.6.3 Digital Health Innovations—But with Equity in Mind

Telehealth platforms offer a fast way to expand mental health support—if designed to reach those on the wrong side of the digital divide. Vouchers for data and devices, bilingual mental health apps, and free 24/7 crisis chat lines could reduce waiting times and empower teens to seek help discreetly (19). However, technology is no silver bullet. Without robust strategies to ensure every disadvantaged child can access and trust these services, digital solutions risk further entrenching inequality rather than alleviating it.

4.7 Conclusion: A Race Against Time to Save a Lost Generation

Britain stands at a pivotal moment, teetering between a path of meaningful reform and a slide into deeper inequity. COVID-19 exposed and magnified the mental health vulnerabilities of our children. If left unaddressed, these psychological wounds may define a generation: permanently blocking some children from realising their potential and cementing a landscape of enduring social inequality.

Yet the crisis also offers a chance to rethink and rebuild. By prioritising mental health in every policy conversation—from education reform to housing and welfare—Britain can prevent the pandemic's emotional fallout from causing lifelong damage. Failure to act decisively means condemning millions of children to carry the pandemic's trauma well into adulthood, perpetuating cycles of poverty, ill health, and despair.

Our children deserve a post-pandemic Britain that invests in their emotional well-being as fiercely as it invests in infrastructure or economic growth. Anything less is a betrayal—one that risks forging a truly lost generation. The question for policymakers, educators, and community leaders is brutally simple: will we choose to protect children's minds and futures, or will we relegate the mental health epidemic to a footnote in the annals of COVID-19?

References

1. World Health Organization (WHO). Depression and other common mental disorders: global health estimates. Geneva: WHO; 2017.
2. Royal College of Psychiatrists. National trends in referral to children and young people's mental health services. London: RCPsych; 2019.
3. Marmot M, Goldblatt P, Allen J, Boyce T, McNeish D, Grady M, et al. Fair society, healthy lives (The Marmot Review). London: UCL Institute of Health Equity; 2010.
4. Department for Education. Special educational needs in England, 2021. London: DfE; 2021.
5. Children's Society. The good childhood report. London: The Children's Society; 2020.
6. Mental Health Foundation. Coronavirus: the divergence of mental health experiences during the pandemic. London: MHF; 2021.
7. Green F. Schoolwork in lockdown: new evidence on the epidemic of educational poverty. LLAKES; 2020.
8. Office for National Statistics (ONS). Coronavirus and the social impacts on Great Britain. London: ONS; 2020.
9. Public Health England (PHE). Disparities in the risk and outcomes of COVID-19. London: PHE; 2020.
10. McMellon C, MacLachlan A. Young people's rights and mental health during a pandemic: an analysis of the impact of emergency legislation in Scotland. YOUNG. 2021 Sep 29:S11–34.
11. Special Needs Jungle. COVID-19 and SEND: the experiences of families. Surrey: SNJ; 2021.
12. The Children's Society. Hidden from view: the experiences of young carers in England. London: The Children's Society; 2013.

13. Stonewall. The school report 2017: the experiences of lesbian, gay, bi and trans young people in Britain's schools. London: Stonewall; 2017.
14. Singh S, Roy D, Sinha K, Parveen S, Sharma G, Joshi G.. Impact of COVID-19 and lockdown on mental health of children and adolescents: a narrative review with recommendations. Psychiatry Res. 2020;293:113429.
15. Shonkoff JP, Garner AS. The lifelong effects of early childhood adversity and toxic stress. Pediatrics. 2012;129(1):e232–46.
16. Centre for Global Development. Learning loss and student dropouts during the COVID-19 pandemic: a review of the evidence two years after schools shut down. Washington (DC): CGDev; 2022.
17. NHS Digital. Mental health of children and young people in England, 2020. Leeds: NHS Digital; 2020.
18. Stevenson C, Wakefield JRH, Felsner I, Drury J, Costa S. Collectively coping with coronavirus: local community identification predicts giving support and lockdown adherence during the COVID-19 pandemic. Br J Soc Psychol. 2021 May 10;60(4).
19. Mental Health Europe. Tele-mental health: guidelines and best practices. Brussels: MHE; 2021.

5 Child Subdemographics

Introduction

The COVID-19 pandemic has proven to be more than just a public health crisis. It has served as a lens magnifying existing social, economic, and health inequities, especially for children whose specific identities or life circumstances confer additional vulnerabilities. In Britain and across the globe, ethnic minority children, LGBTQ+ youth, young carers, asylum seekers, and children with disabilities have often experienced a "double burden": first, grappling with the universal challenges of the pandemic (such as school closures, social isolation, reduced access to healthcare), and second, contending with barriers that reflect entrenched discrimination and systemic neglect.

The overarching aim of this chapter is to examine these intersecting dimensions of disadvantage and the consequent health impacts on various groups of children during the COVID-19 pandemic. "Health" here is understood in the broad, holistic sense championed by the World Health Organization—encompassing physical, mental, and social well-being. Using an intersectionality framework, this chapter explores how overlapping identities (e.g., ethnicity, sexual orientation, disability status, and caring responsibilities) shaped experiences of the pandemic, determined access to resources, and, ultimately, altered the trajectory of childhood health.

The discussion begins by establishing key conceptual underpinnings, including the notion of intersectionality and social determinants of health in a pandemic context. It then delves into the pandemic's effects on children from ethnic minority backgrounds, LGBTQ+ youth, children with disabilities, young carers, children in the asylum system, and other marginalised groups. The chapter concludes by highlighting potential policy and community-level interventions to mitigate these health disparities and offers a forward-looking perspective on how we might harness the lessons of COVID-19 to develop more inclusive, resilient systems of support for vulnerable children.

DOI: 10.4324/9781003312529-6

5.1 Conceptual Foundations: Intersectionality and Social Determinants of Health

5.1.1 *Intersectionality and Child Health*

Originally conceptualised by Kimberlé Crenshaw (1), intersectionality emphasises how social identities—such as race, gender, sexual orientation, disability, or class—interact to shape unique experiences of privilege or disadvantage. Within the context of child health, an intersectional lens facilitates deeper insights into why some groups of children have been disproportionately impacted by the pandemic. For instance, a young carer from an ethnic minority background living in a deprived neighbourhood faces a confluence of risk factors that differ markedly from those of a child who shares only one of those identities.

By centring intersectionality, this chapter advocates for moving beyond siloed approaches that consider "children" as a monolith and, instead, calls for nuanced understandings of how health outcomes are patterned by multiple overlapping identities. This approach is particularly salient in a pandemic context, wherein existing inequalities often become both more visible and more severe (2).

5.1.2 *Social Determinants of Health in a Pandemic Context*

The social determinants of health—income, education, housing, neighbourhood conditions, and social support networks—play an integral role in dictating health outcomes (3). During the pandemic, these determinants became even more pronounced:

- Housing: Overcrowded, poor-quality housing increased the risk of infection and complicated self-isolation measures for many families, particularly among disadvantaged communities (4).
- Digital Divide: Access to technology proved pivotal once education, social services, and even mental health support moved online. Children from low-income families and marginalised groups often found themselves digitally excluded, with adverse consequences for both education and well-being (5).
- Social Capital: Lockdowns and social distancing disproportionately affected children reliant on informal community or extended family networks for emotional, mental, and cultural support.

Taken together, these social determinants, when filtered through the lens of intersectionality, help explain why certain child populations experienced worse health outcomes, deeper learning losses, and heightened stress during COVID-19.

5.2   Ethnic Minority Children and the Disproportionate Burden of COVID-19

5.2.1   *Pre-Pandemic Disparities and Structural Racism*

Long before the emergence of COVID-19, ethnic minority children in the UK faced systemic obstacles: higher levels of poverty, ongoing experiences of racism, and underfunded schools serving communities of colour (6). Public Health England's review of disparities in COVID-19 outcomes reaffirmed a well-documented trend: individuals from Black, Asian, and other minority ethnic backgrounds generally had worse morbidity and mortality rates from the virus (7). These disparities were not genetic inevitabilities but the product of intersecting socioeconomic and structural factors, including greater likelihood of living in multi-generational households, working in high-exposure frontline occupations, and having limited access to timely healthcare.

For children specifically, the fear and anxiety surrounding infections in the household amplified stress. Parents who worked in essential jobs often could not "shield", leaving families more vulnerable to exposure. Additionally, the closure or reduction of community-specific social support services (e.g., faith-based youth groups, cultural associations) stripped away crucial networks that mitigate daily stress and racial discrimination (8).

5.2.2   *Educational Disruption and Widening Achievement Gaps*

Ethnic minority children were also disproportionately affected by school closures and the shift to remote learning. A 2021 study by the Education Policy Institute found that pupils from Black and Bangladeshi backgrounds faced comparatively higher digital exclusion, lacking the necessary devices or internet connections to participate in online classes (9). This was further compounded by language barriers in some households, limiting parents' capacity to assist with home-based learning.

While some minority ethnic groups had been bridging educational gaps prior to the pandemic, COVID-19 triggered regressions in attainment for many. The intersection of poverty, racism, and digital exclusion crystallised in tangible ways, with some studies suggesting that the most socioeconomically deprived minority ethnic students could be an additional 2–3 months behind their peers (10).

5.2.3   *Mental Health Strains*

Mental health ramifications were especially significant for ethnic minority youth, who sometimes reported heightened racial tensions during lockdown (11). Anecdotal reports from community organisations also pointed to increased instances of racist bullying in online settings, where anonymity can embolden hateful behaviour (12). Without in-person school communities—where teachers might intervene—these incidents sometimes went unaddressed.

Furthermore, the pandemic context that labelled COVID-19 as a "foreign virus" (with certain media outlets stigmatising Asians in particular) heightened experiences of discrimination (13). Children from East or Southeast Asian backgrounds reported fear and isolation, at times feeling unable to voice these fears in largely white school environments. The cumulative effect of racism, fear of illness, and economic insecurity weighed heavily on mental health.

5.2.4   Lessons and Avenues for Addressing Disparities

Addressing the pandemic's disproportionate impact on ethnic minority children demands systemic responses:

- Equitable Health Outreach: Targeted testing, vaccination drives, and culturally sensitive public health messaging can reduce both stigma and infection rates in marginalised communities (7).
- Digital Inclusion Strategies: Policy measures ensuring free or heavily subsidised digital access for low-income ethnic minority households could alleviate educational setbacks (5).
- Anti-Racist School Policies: Schools should enact zero-tolerance approaches to racist bullying in virtual as well as physical contexts, accompanied by staff training on how racism intersects with the pandemic.
- Community Partnerships: Collaborations with local faith institutions, cultural organisations, and ethnic minority-led charities can strengthen trust and facilitate more effective mental health support for children (14).

5.3   LGBTQ+ Youth: Isolation, Identity, and Health Challenges

5.3.1   Pre-Existing Vulnerabilities

LGBTQ+ young people often face a precarious environment in schools, homes, and broader society, contending with stigma and, in many cases, bullying (15). They are already at higher risk of poor mental health, self-harm, and suicide attempts compared to their heterosexual, cisgender peers (16). During COVID-19, the closure of schools and youth centres—and the enforced confinement to home environments that might be unaccepting—intensified these vulnerabilities.

5.3.2   Loss of Affirming Spaces

For many LGBTQ+ children, in-person contact with supportive peers, LGBTQ+ youth groups, or inclusive school clubs is essential for maintaining self-esteem and emotional well-being (17). The pandemic abruptly halted these face-to-face interactions. Although some organisations shifted to online support, children lacking private internet access or whose parents monitored their digital usage often could not participate freely.

Moreover, homeschooling in unsupportive families subjected some LGBTQ+ youths to misgendering, derogatory remarks, or denial of their identity on a near-constant basis. Mental health hotlines (like Childline in the UK) reported a spike in calls from young people grappling with sexuality- or gender-related distress during lockdown (18).

5.3.3   Delayed or Denied Gender-Affirming Healthcare

Transgender and gender-questioning children faced acute challenges when healthcare and counselling services were deprioritised or postponed as a result of the pandemic's strain on the NHS. Appointments at gender identity clinics, which already had lengthy waiting times, were often cancelled or delayed (19). The heightened dysphoria and uncertainty exacerbated depression, anxiety, and risk of self-harm.

Additionally, restrictions on physical activity, such as swimming or sports, removed valuable outlets for bodily expression and stress relief for some transgender youth. This confluence of medical and social pressures magnified the emotional toll.

5.3.4   Online Risks and Opportunities

While remote and digital platforms often provided lifelines for connecting with LGBTQ+ allies, they also introduced risks. Cyberbullying rose in some cases, with homophobic and transphobic harassment going unchecked (20). Additionally, spending more time online could expose young people to harmful content if they lacked robust guidance or digital literacy.

Nevertheless, some LGBTQ+ youth discovered supportive online communities—chat groups, gaming platforms, social media movements—where they forged friendships and accessed advice. Thus, digital spaces functioned as a double-edged sword: enabling vital connection for some while precipitating new forms of victimisation for others.

5.3.5   Emerging Solutions for LGBTQ+ Youth

A supportive post-pandemic landscape for LGBTQ+ children requires:

- Enhanced Access to Mental Health Services: Telehealth programmes specialised in LGBTQ+ issues can mitigate challenges linked to waiting times and geographic location.

- Safer Online Environments: School administrators and social media platforms should strengthen anti-hate policies, ensuring swift responses to cyberbullying.
- Inclusive Education Policies: Mandating LGBTQ+ content in sex and relationship education helps build a more tolerant peer environment (21).
- Gender-Affirming Healthcare Pathways: Adequate funding and resource prioritisation for transgender-specific services is critical for preventing further deterioration in mental health.

5.4 Children with Disabilities: Heightened Vulnerabilities

5.4.1 Pre-Pandemic Marginalisation

Children with disabilities—be they physical, intellectual, or developmental—often encounter a healthcare and education system ill-equipped to meet their needs. Many depend on specialised interventions, therapies, and support workers to maintain functional independence and cope with everyday activities (22). When these services were interrupted by COVID-19 restrictions, families scrambled to provide care independently, often without training or respite.

5.4.2 Disruption of Essential Services

Occupational therapy, speech and language therapy, physiotherapy, and social care visits were severely curtailed or moved online during lockdowns (23). Virtual therapy often proved insufficient for children with complex communication needs or sensory processing disorders. The regression in motor skills, language abilities, and academic attainment in some disabled children was significant, threatening long-term development.

Special schools or integrated programmes that offered crucial social interaction, structured routines, and targeted learning support were closed to most pupils, except in some cases where they were designated as vulnerable. However, fear of infection sometimes deterred parents from sending children in, given heightened clinical vulnerabilities in certain disabilities.

5.4.3 Mental Health and Caregiver Stress

Children with disabilities often rely on consistent routines to manage anxiety. COVID-19 disrupted these routines, leaving families to manage challenging behaviours, meltdowns, or increased emotional distress without professional assistance (24). Parents and siblings stepped in as de facto carers, leading to burnout and exacerbating mental health struggles across entire households.

For those with learning disabilities, the closure of day centres and respite services removed vital forms of stimulation and socialisation. Such isolation fuelled a rise in mental health issues, including depression and loneliness (25).

Meanwhile, practical concerns—such as ensuring continuity of medication supplies—also created additional burdens.

5.4.4   *Bridging the Gap for Disabled Children*

Improved planning and resources are crucial to safeguarding children with disabilities in times of crisis:

- Continuity of Therapy: Prioritising in-person or well-designed telehealth services for essential therapies could mitigate regression in developmental progress (22).
- Adaptive Equipment and Technology: Greater investment in accessible technology (e.g., augmentative and alternative communication devices) can ensure that disabled children remain engaged in remote education (26).
- Caregiver Support: Expanding short-break or respite provisions, even during public health emergencies, eases family stress.
- Inclusive Policy Planning: Actively consulting disabled people's organisations and families when designing pandemic responses can prevent inadvertent neglect of their needs.

5.5   Young Carers: Bearing Adult Responsibilities in a Pandemic

5.5.1   *Defining Young Carers*

Young carers are children and adolescents who provide unpaid care for a family member—often a parent or sibling—who might be experiencing chronic illness, disability, mental health challenges, or addiction (27). Even before COVID-19, these youths faced pressures that impinged upon their educational performance, social life, and emotional well-being.

5.5.2   *Lockdowns and Increased Caring Responsibilities*

During the pandemic, the burden on young carers escalated drastically. With lockdowns curtailing external care visits and shutting down day centres, young carers had to shoulder greater responsibilities, including administering medication, providing personal care, managing household tasks, and offering emotional support (28). This expanded caregiving role, coupled with remote schooling, was immensely stressful.

Moreover, many young carers lost crucial respite opportunities—after-school clubs, meeting friends, or simply having time away from home. The combination of academic demands and caregiving left them exhausted, with little space for self-care or normal childhood experiences.

5.5.3 Educational and Social Setbacks

Remote learning often proved untenable for young carers needing to juggle domestic tasks. Attendance and engagement in online classes waned, resulting in significant learning loss (29). Teachers sometimes misunderstood or overlooked the extent of caregiving demands, offering little leeway for missed assignments or absent "attendance" in virtual sessions.

Social isolation was yet another challenge. Young carers often experience limited peer networks under normal circumstances; lockdown only heightened their seclusion. Lacking robust social support, many faced deteriorating mental health, with some studies indicating elevated rates of anxiety and depression among young carers (30).

5.5.4 Policy and Practice Recommendations

To safeguard the well-being of young carers during public health crises, policymakers, and institutions should:

Identify and Support: Enhanced screening and clear referral pathways in schools, GP surgeries, and social services can help locate young carers early (31).

- Flexible Schooling: Tailored schedules, extended deadlines, and additional tutoring support can ensure that caregiving duties do not derail educational progress.
- Respite Services: Even in lockdown conditions, creative solutions (such as short virtual respite programmes) could offer moments of relief.
- Financial Assistance: Families reliant on a child's caregiving labour may require targeted financial support or additional social care services to mitigate the need for intensive child involvement (28).

5.6 Asylum-Seeking and Refugee Children: Precarity and Isolation

5.6.1 Already on the Margins

Asylum-seeking and refugee children enter the UK under precarious, often traumatic circumstances. They may arrive unaccompanied or with family members equally vulnerable. Language barriers, uncertain immigration status, and limited financial resources frequently conspire to create extreme disadvantage (32).

5.6.2 COVID-19 Impacts: Shelter, Healthcare, and Legal Support

During the pandemic, asylum seekers in cramped government accommodation struggled to maintain social distancing (33). Limited English proficiency impeded access to up-to-date health information, while fear of deportation dissuaded some from seeking medical help. For refugee children with complex post-traumatic stress disorder (PTSD), abrupt changes in service provision—a shift to online counselling or suspended in-person therapy—complicated mental health support (34).

Furthermore, the closure of legal aid clinics and in-person interpretation services stalled many asylum claims, perpetuating the stress of indefinite waiting. Children, already grappling with disrupted education, faced additional uncertainty around their future, exacerbating anxiety and compounding other negative health determinants.

5.6.3   Educational Barriers

Remote schooling proved exceptionally challenging for refugee children lacking stable internet access, personal devices, or language support (35). In households where multiple children required a single device, conflicts over usage were common. Some asylum-seeking families, living on minimal allowances, simply could not afford broadband. Consequently, many refugee children experienced an abrupt cessation of formal education, risking long-term academic setbacks.

5.6.4   Future Directions for Refugee Child Health

- Secure, Decent Housing: Minimising crowding and ensuring safe accommodation can reduce infection risks and provide a stable environment for children to study.
- Culturally Competent Healthcare: Medical and mental health professionals trained in cultural awareness and trauma-informed practices are essential for addressing the complex needs of refugee children (33).
- Language Access: Schools and local authorities can invest in bilingual teaching assistants, interpreters, and translated educational materials to facilitate smoother remote or blended learning.
- Legal Safeguards: Streamlined asylum processes and protected legal routes for unaccompanied minors can alleviate the psychological burden of uncertainty.

5.7   Other Marginalised Groups: Rural Isolation, Homeless Children, and More

5.7.1   Rural Children

Children living in remote or rural areas often encountered additional hurdles during the pandemic. Limited broadband infrastructure inhibited remote learning, while lengthy distances from healthcare facilities complicated access to

COVID-19 testing, paediatric care, and mental health services (36). Youth in rural communities also faced social isolation, as youth clubs or extracurricular activities were restricted.

5.7.2 Homeless and Temporarily Housed Children

Families experiencing homelessness or living in temporary accommodation struggled to comply with lockdown protocols. Overcrowded hostels or B&Bs (bed and breakfasts) made self-isolation or home schooling nearly impossible. Loss of in-person support (e.g., from homeless shelters or charities) heightened food insecurity and mental distress (37). Children in such unstable living conditions faced disruptions to schooling, intensifying educational and social marginalisation.

5.7.3 Children in the Care System

Looked-after children—those under local authority care—also faced specific upheavals during COVID-19. Foster carers reported increased strain due to home learning, while contact with birth families was disrupted or moved online, raising concerns about attachment and emotional well-being (38). Some care leavers encountered precarious financial circumstances when part-time work dried up, with limited recourse to public funds.

5.8 Policy Responses and Community Innovations

5.8.1 Government Interventions and Their Shortfalls

Across the UK, governments introduced measures intended to protect vulnerable children during the pandemic: free school meal vouchers, the "Everyone In" policy for rough sleepers, increased Universal Credit, and digital device distribution in schools (39). While each measure provided partial relief, structural deficits and inconsistent rollouts meant that many children—especially those at the intersections of disadvantage—slipped through the cracks.

5.8.2 Grassroots and Community-Led Solutions

Local charities, mutual aid groups, and faith-based organisations played pivotal roles in offering direct support to marginalised children (40). From delivering laptops and meals to providing mental health hotlines in multiple languages, these grassroots endeavours often responded more swiftly and adaptively than centralised agencies. Their limitations, however, lay in capacity and funding uncertainties, emphasising the need for sustained public investment in community infrastructures.

5.8.3 Harnessing Digital Innovations

The pandemic accelerated the adoption of telehealth and remote counselling services for children, including LGBTQ+-specific virtual clinics, mental health chatlines for young carers, and video-based language tutoring for refugee children (41). These models, if refined and supported post-pandemic, could become permanent fixtures in bridging service gaps—particularly for those in rural areas or with limited mobility. Nevertheless, bridging the digital divide remains a prerequisite for equitable access.

5.8.4 Building on Intersectional Policy Frameworks

Moving forward, an intersectional approach must be woven into all levels of policy design:

- Data Disaggregation: Collecting data by race, disability status, sexual orientation (where appropriate for age), and migration status can illuminate specific vulnerabilities and target interventions more effectively.
- Cross-Sector Collaboration: Health, education, and social care agencies must share data and strategies to safeguard children holistically.
- Representation: Involving children and young people from affected groups in policymaking ensures that interventions are co-designed with, rather than imposed upon, those most in need.

5.9 Looking Beyond COVID-19: Towards Resilience and Equity

5.9.1 The Long Shadow of the Pandemic

For many children in vulnerable demographics, the pandemic's impacts will reverberate for years—if not decades. Learning loss, mental health strains, lost family members, and increased poverty rates are likely to shape adolescence and early adulthood, potentially entrenching cycles of marginalisation. Researchers' project that health inequities widened under COVID-19 could lead to a surge in chronic conditions, mental health crises, and diminished socioeconomic prospects (42).

5.9.2 A Window of Opportunity

Despite the severe challenges, the pandemic has illuminated what truly matters: the vital role of community solidarity, the capacity for rapid policy shifts, and the need for robust social safety nets. Stakeholders now possess an unprecedented impetus to rectify long-standing inequities. If governments, nonprofits, and private sector entities harness this momentum, the post-pandemic reconstruction could generate more equitable, resilient systems.

5.9.3 Recommendations for a More Equitable Future

1. **Guaranteed Minimum Standards of Digital Access**
   Mandating universal internet connectivity and device provision for low-income families would help ensure continuity of education and health services, especially under future crises.
2. **Ring-Fenced Funding for Marginalised Groups**
   Specific funding pots—earmarked for ethnic minority communities, LGBTQ+ youth, disabled children, and young carers—could guarantee that additional needs are not overshadowed by more general recovery strategies.
3. **Strengthening Child-Centred Infrastructure**
   Investing in children's centres, youth clubs, and school-based mental health services addresses both the immediate aftermath of COVID-19 and fosters community resilience.
4. **Multilayered Inclusion in Pandemic Preparedness**

Lessons learned should be embedded in future emergency planning, ensuring that children's voices and diverse experiences inform contingency protocols for schooling, healthcare, and community support.

5.9.4 Conclusion

The COVID-19 pandemic has been a crucible, exposing long-standing fault lines of inequality in the UK and worldwide. Ethnic minority children, LGBTQ+ youth, children with disabilities, young carers, and other marginalised groups have borne an outsized share of the pandemic's hardships, with negative repercussions for their physical health, mental well-being, and educational progress. Yet crises can also drive structural reform.

The real challenge lies in translating the harsh lessons of COVID-19 into transformative policy changes that secure and expand the rights and well-being of every child—regardless of background or identity. By embracing intersectionality, championing inclusive policy design, and investing in community-led innovations, society can begin to address both the immediate fallout of the pandemic and the deeper inequities it revealed. Only through such a holistic and equitable approach can we ensure that, when the next crisis comes, no child is left to bear disproportionate burdens.

References

1. Crenshaw KW. Demarginalizing the intersection of race and sex: a black feminist critique of antidiscrimination doctrine, feminist theory and anti-racist politics. Univ Chic Leg Forum. 1989;139–67.
2. Bambra C, Riordan R, Ford J, Matthews F. The COVID-19 pandemic and health inequalities. J Epidemiol Community Health. 2020;74(11):964–8.

3. Marmot M, Goldblatt P, Allen J, Boyce T, McNeish D, Grady M, et al. Fair society, healthy lives (The Marmot Review). London: UCL Institute of Health Equity; 2010.
4. Department for Levelling Up, Housing & Communities. English housing survey 2020–21: headline report. London: DLUHC; 2022.
5. Green F. Schoolwork in lockdown: new evidence on the epidemic of educational poverty. LLAKES; 2020.
6. Equality and Human Rights Commission (EHRC). Race report: healing a divided Britain. London: EHRC; 2016.
7. Public Health England (PHE). Disparities in the risk and outcomes of COVID-19. London: PHE; 2020.
8. Nazroo J, Bécares L. Ethnic inequalities in COVID-19 mortality: a consequence of persistent racism. Runnymede Trust; 2021.
9. Education Policy Institute (EPI). Education in England: annual report 2021. London: EPI; 2021.
10. Reay D. Miseducation: inequality, education and the working classes. Bristol: Policy Press; 2017.
11. Public Health England. Beyond the data: Understanding the impact of COVID-19 on BAME Groups; 2020.
12. McMellon C, MacLachlan A. Young people's rights and mental health during a pandemic: an analysis of the impact of emergency legislation in Scotland. YOUNG. 2021 Sep 29:S11–34.
13. Li Y, Nicholson HL. When "model minorities" become "yellow peril"— othering and the racialisation of Asian Americans in the COVID-19 pandemic. Sociol Compass. 2021;15:e12849.
14. Nuffield Foundation. COVID realities: documenting life on a low income during the pandemic. London: Nuffield Foundation; 2021.
15. Stonewall. The school report 2017: the experiences of lesbian, gay, bi and trans young people in Britain's schools. London: Stonewall; 2017.
16. McDermott E, Hughes E, Rawlings V. The social determinants of lesbian, gay, bisexual and trans youth suicidality in England: a mixed methods study. J Public Health (Oxf). 2017;40(3):e244–51.
17. Meyer IH. Prejudice, social stress, and mental health in lesbian, gay, and bisexual populations: conceptual issues and research evidence. Psychol Bull. 2003;129(5):674–97.
18. Childline. Childline annual review: the impact of COVID-19 on children and young people. London: NSPCC; 2021.
19. NHS England. Gender dysphoria services: data on waiting times. London: NHS; 2021.
20. Suzannah Allkins. Online safety: The impact of the coronavirus pandemic on children in the UK. J Fam Child Health. 2021.
21. Department for Education. Relationships, sex and health education guidance. London: DfE; 2019.
22. Special Needs Jungle. COVID-19 and SEND: the experiences of families. SNJ; 2021.
23. Royal College of Occupational Therapists. The impact of COVID-19 on occupational therapy services for children. London: RCOT; 2020.

24. Carers UK. Caring behind closed doors: six months on. London: Carers UK; 2020.
25. Mencap. Impact of COVID-19 on people with a learning disability. London: Mencap; 2021.
26. Department for Digital, Culture, Media & Sport. The UK digital strategy. London: DCMS; 2022.
27. The Children's Society. Hidden from view: the experiences of young carers in England. London: The Children's Society; 2013.
28. Carers Trust. Supporting young carers in schools programme. London: Carers Trust; 2020.
29. Hayes D, Fancourt D, Burton A. The experiences and impact of the COVID-19 pandemic on young carers: practice implications and planning for future health emergencies. Child Adolesc Psychiatry Ment Health. 2024 Jan 3;18(1).
30. Scotland's Commissioner for Children and Young People. Lockdown lowdown: the impact of COVID-19 on children in Scotland. Edinburgh: SCCYP; 2020.
31. Wong S. Young carers in the NHS. Br J Gen Pract. 2017 Oct 26;67(664):527–8.
32. Refugee Council. Children in the asylum system. London: Refugee Council; 2021.
33. Doctors of the World UK. An unsafe distance: the impact of COVID-19 on asylum seekers in the UK. London: DOTW; 2020.
34. Meyer SR, Robinson WC, Chhim S, Bass J. Labour migration and mental health in Cambodia: a qualitative study. Int J Ment Health Syst. 2020;14(1):72. [NB: Example global perspective of refugee/forced migration mental health.]
35. Coronavirus and the impact of school closures on refugees and asylum seekers in the United Kingdom. International Migration Research Network (IMISCOE); 2020.
36. DEFRA. Rural populations and broadband connectivity: policy update. London: DEFRA; 2020.
37. Shelter. Homelessness in a pandemic: impact on families and children. London: Shelter; 2021.
38. Department for Education. Children looked after in England including adoptions, 2020/21. London: DfE; 2021.
39. HM Government. COVID-19 winter plan: support for vulnerable families. London: HM Government; 2021.
40. Stevenson C, Wakefield JRH, Felsner I, Drury J, Costa S. Collectively coping with coronavirus: Local community identification predicts giving support and lockdown adherence during the COVID-19 pandemic. Br J Soc Psychol. 2021 May 10;60(4).
41. YoungMinds. Coronavirus: impact on young people with mental health needs. London: YoungMinds; 2021.
42. Bambra C, Lynch J, Smith KE. The unequal pandemic: COVID-19 and health inequalities. Bristol: Policy Press; 2021.

6   Wider Implications

Introduction

Britain stands at a crossroads. While the country has long touted itself as a
global leader in social welfare and healthcare, a closer look at children's living conditions reveals glaring disparities—what many researchers call "health
inequities" rather than mere "differences" (1). The plight of disadvantaged
children, if left unaddressed, reverberates throughout the adult population
and into old age, undermining social cohesion, eroding trust in institutions,
and exerting unsustainable pressure on public finances. In short, ignoring
child health inequities creates a cascade of social and economic crises that no
one—young, middle-aged, or elderly—can evade indefinitely.

This chapter ventures beyond well-trodden ground to probe less-explored
terrain: namely, how a child's ill health or deprivation in early life sows hidden
turbulence for working adults and older populations. We will unpack how these
inequities compromise Britain's social fabric and undermine the nation's economic
resilience. Far from a narrow "charity case", child health equity is a moral and
pragmatic imperative with ripple effects that shape the destiny of every generation.

In weaving together findings from diverse fields—public health, economics, sociology, and mental health research—we reveal a stark truth: a society
that permits its youngest citizens to fall behind is essentially mortgaging its
future, incurring steep costs in healthcare, lost productivity, and social disin-
tegration (2,3). This story, bolstered by data from PubMed-indexed sources,
is a clarion call for radical reform and a recalibration of collective priorities.
The survival of the welfare state, the intergenerational contract, and Britain's
competitive edge depends on whether the country can muster the resolve to
eliminate child health inequities at their roots.

6.1   Child Health Inequities: A Threat That Spares No One

6.1.1   The Broader Definition of "Health"

In discussing child health, we must adopt the expansive definition championed by the World Health Organization (WHO), which views health as

DOI: 10.4324/9781003312529-7

encompassing physical, mental, and social well-being (4). Childhood obesity, chronic respiratory infections, lack of immunisation, and inadequate mental health support represent only the visible tip of a much bigger iceberg of disadvantage. The literature underscores that such inequities form early and deepen over time, adversely shaping not only physical growth but also educational attainment, emotional development, and social integration (5).

Although such disparities have persisted for decades, the COVID-19 pandemic drew fresh attention to them. A 2021 systematic review in The Lancet Child & Adolescent Health reported that children from socioeconomically disadvantaged backgrounds faced more severe disruptions in schooling, nutrition, and mental health services during lockdowns (6). The tragedy is not that we lack the knowledge to address these problems; it is that the cumulative social cost of ignoring them remains underappreciated.

6.1.2 Child Health: A Foreshadowing of National Fortunes

Children are the generational scaffolding upon which a nation builds its future. Robust child health signals a vibrant pipeline of future workers, consumers, innovators, and caregivers. Conversely, inequities in child well-being—be it through preventable diseases, malnutrition, or mental distress—constitute a ticking time bomb for the entire society (7). Studies consistently show that children struggling with chronic conditions or emotional trauma are more likely to underperform academically, enter adulthood without stable employment, and experience higher rates of morbidity and mortality (8).

A large-scale birth cohort analysis from PubMed found that childhood adversity—spanning poverty, abuse, and inadequate healthcare—heightens the risk of metabolic syndrome, cardiovascular disease, and mental illness in later life (9). When multiplied across millions of individuals, these personal health trajectories weigh heavily on tax revenues, the NHS, and the economy's productive capacity. In short, no adult or elder can escape the indirect fiscal and social consequences of a neglected childhood population.

6.2 Impact on Working Adults: Spiralling Economic and Emotional Costs

6.2.1 The "Hidden" Burden on Caregivers

For many families, a child's health crisis triggers a relentless cycle of missed workdays, lost income, and stunted career trajectories. This dynamic is particularly devastating for single parents, though dual-earner households are not immune. A child grappling with severe asthma (exacerbated by damp, mouldy housing) or with an unaddressed mental health issue may require frequent appointments and at-home supervision. In a systematic review available on PubMed, parents reported heightened stress, reduced work productivity, and potential job loss when faced with recurrent child health problems, especially in under-resourced neighbourhoods with few social supports (10).

The long-term cost to the adult's emotional well-being is staggering. Chronic stress fosters a higher risk of depression and anxiety, which further erodes parental functioning. According to an article in Social Psychiatry and Psychiatric Epidemiology, parents of chronically ill children exhibited almost twice the prevalence of depressive symptoms compared with parents whose children had no major health complaints (11). Unable to cope, they often cut back on working hours or exit the labour force, dragging down household earnings and tax contributions.

6.2.2   *Workplace Disruption and Lost Productivity*

From the employer's standpoint, child health inequities among employees' families translate into increased absenteeism, lower morale, and frequent staff turnover. A Journal of Occupational and Environmental Medicine article documents the financial burden companies shoulder when staff frequently take leave to care for sick children (12). Over time, these disruptions can also lower workplace innovation and teamwork, especially in smaller firms that lack robust parental support policies.

Moreover, a workforce reeling from child-focused stress can become less receptive to training opportunities, less adaptive to market changes, and less creative. The net effect is a slow but inexorable decline in the firm's competitiveness, an outcome mirrored across the economy if child health inequity proliferates widely. Hence, the damage is not limited to individual families: entire industries can falter, undermining Britain's reputation as an economic powerhouse.

6.2.3   *Emotional Spillover: From Home to Community*

Beyond financial strain, the psychological toll of caring for a disadvantaged or chronically unwell child often spills over into community life. Exhausted, overwhelmed parents might withdraw from local civic activities—such as volunteering, neighbourhood committees, or supporting local schools—further weakening the social fabric. This disconnection intensifies in lower-income areas, where public amenities are already inadequate. As a result, the local "middle ground" of social life erodes, making communities more susceptible to social isolation, distrust, and conflict. In essence, allowing child health inequities to fester shrinks the capacity of adults to engage in the communal sphere, fracturing the solidarity needed for a healthy democracy.

6.3   The Elderly: Bearing the Shockwaves of Childhood Deprivation

6.3.1   *Intergenerational Dependencies*

An ageing population depends upon a robust, healthy, and skilled younger generation to sustain pension funds, social services, and healthcare provisions.

environment but also the long-term stability of a country's social fabric. Child health inequities signify deep-rooted structural problems, signalling to foreign investors that the country might suffer heightened healthcare costs, social unrest, and policy volatility. This can deter inward investment, further constraining economic expansion.

Domestically, more citizens lose faith in the political establishment's willingness or ability to tackle fundamental injustices. Anti-elite or populist sentiments flourish when large groups feel abandoned by a system that invests too little in childhood development. As these groups gain traction, policy predictability wanes, and business uncertainty climbs, compounding the economic disadvantages of widespread child health inequities.

6.5 Social Cohesion in Jeopardy: Child Health Inequity as a Catalyst for Division

6.5.1 Eroding Trust and Rising Polarisation

In many British communities, particularly post-industrial areas or impoverished rural pockets, child health inequities become visible in school absenteeism, hunger, mental distress, and juvenile crime. Observers blame parents, local councils, the national government, or "the system", creating a mosaic of finger-pointing rather than solutions. Over time, this fosters a climate of polarisation. Those who remain untouched by these hardships grow resentful of increased taxes or welfare policies, while struggling communities feel scapegoated. Tensions mount as the "us vs. them" narrative intensifies—a direct blow to the concept of national unity (18).

6.5.2 The Pathway to Deviance and Crime

Research in criminology, including PubMed-indexed longitudinal studies, suggests that repeated experiences of deprivation and neglect can steer adolescents into deviant activities (19). This pathway is neither deterministic nor universally applicable, but the likelihood grows when a child's basic needs for stable housing, proper nutrition, and supportive adult relationships remain unmet. Gangs or extremist ideologies often promise an alternative sense of identity, respect, or economic gain absent in mainstream settings. The eventual costs to society—through policing, courts, and prisons—far surpass what early child health and social investments would have cost.

6.5.3 Fragmented Communities and Shallow Solidarity

Generations that have grown up witnessing persistent child health inequities in their neighbourhoods often internalise a narrative of systemic abandonment. They disengage from local institutions—youth clubs, community centres, or the local political process—because they see no tangible benefit. Once civic engagement flags, everything from litter to petty crime can spike, as communal efforts to maintain a safe, clean environment crumble. The intangible sense of belonging that once held communities together dissolves, leaving behind an echo of cynicism and frustration.

6.6   A Cultural and Moral Crisis: Britain's Identity at Stake

6.6.1   Undermining the Tradition of Compassion

British society has long championed itself for institutional compassion—welfare states, universal healthcare, and robust public education. But child health inequities starkly reveal the gap between ideals and lived reality. If significant numbers of children cannot access timely medical care, adequate nutrition, or safe environments, the mythos of Britain as a fair and benevolent society rings hollow. The disillusionment is felt not merely by the disadvantaged families but also by well-meaning citizens dismayed to see their nation failing its youngest.

6.6.2   Shrinking Global Soft Power

Soft power—a nation's ability to sway international affairs through cultural influence, moral authority, and humanitarian leadership—depends in part on demonstrating internal coherence and social justice. The country that bungles its child health outcomes projects inconsistency, potentially undermining its standing in global dialogues on human rights, poverty reduction, or global health (20). International partners may question Britain's credibility or be less inclined to collaborate on projects requiring mutual trust in social commitments. Hence, the moral crisis at home constrains the UK's capacity to lead abroad.

6.6.3   Undervalued Human Capital

From an anthropological perspective, children are carriers of cultural continuity—future guardians of heritage, language, and social norms. When health inequities curtail their potential, we also lose intangible cultural capital. Britain's arts, sports, research, and social institutions all thrive on new generations pushing boundaries. A 2019 PubMed article underscored the importance of "youthful innovation" in perpetuating cultural and scientific breakthroughs (21). Blocking that innovation through neglect or underinvestment is a collective folly that jeopardises Britain's legacy and global contributions.

6.7 Taking Responsibility: Why You Should Care, Even If You're "Safe"

6.7.1 No Geographical Escape

Some might presume that residing in affluent communities insulates them from the ravages of child health inequities. Yet new forms of social and financial interconnectivity mean no region stands entirely alone. Surges in community-level healthcare costs eventually balloon national insurance rates, and local workforce shortages hamper the supply chains that feed high-end consumer markets. Moreover, children from disadvantaged backgrounds do not remain static; they may migrate, entering other labour markets or educational institutions, influencing society far beyond their birth locale (22).

6.7.2 The True Economic Price Tag

The tax burden, public spending adjustments, and potential inflationary pressures triggered by neglected youth reverberate in every income bracket. Even private healthcare subscribers or wealthy pensioners have a stake, because significant NHS shortfalls can spur governmental cost-cutting or reallocation of funds, potentially impacting everything from infrastructure to local policing. Ultimately, the notion of "it won't affect me" is a fantasy, undone by the realities of integrated national budgets and overlapping social systems.

6.7.3 Moral Imperatives That Cut Across Politics

Child well-being is a cause that transcends conventional left-right divides. Conservatives can champion early intervention to curtail future welfare dependency and crime costs, while progressives can advocate for the moral and egalitarian grounds that every child deserves equal life chances. Centrists see child health equity as a bulwark against radical social upheaval. In an era of political fragmentation, child well-being might serve as one of the few rallying points that garners broad-based support, offering a unifying narrative for a deeply divided electorate (23).

6.8 Policy Reboot: Strategies to Avert a Multi-Generational Disaster

6.8.1 Universal Early-Years Intervention

Robust evidence shows that interventions in the first 1,000 days of life can yield enormous returns. From in-home nurse visits to nutritional supplements for pregnant women and infants, such efforts drastically reduce the risk of low birth weight, stunting, and early cognitive deficits (24). In Britain, scaling up the Health Visitor Programme or reintroducing children's centres—equipped with multi-agency teams—could close gaps that currently funnel children into a life of ill health and deprivation.

6.8.2   Wrap-Around School Hubs

Schools remain the frontline for detecting childhood adversities and bridging resource gaps. Converting schools into "wrap-around hubs" that provide not only education but also health screenings, mental health counselling, meal programmes, and community outreach can break the cycle of disadvantage (25). Teacher training in trauma-informed practices—backed by social workers and healthcare professionals—ensures that early signs of mental distress or nutritional deficiency are not missed. The cost of hiring additional personnel may be offset by the vast public savings derived from reduced hospital admissions and better-educated, healthier youth.

6.8.3   Housing Overhauls

Substandard housing is a key driver of respiratory illnesses, stress, and unstable family routines. Revising planning regulations, increasing social housing stock, and offering incentives for affordable rentals can ameliorate the pressures that lock children into overcrowded, damp environments (26). A 2020 PubMed-indexed cross-sectional study in the UK found significant associations between damp housing and paediatric respiratory admissions, with children in the lowest income quintile disproportionately affected (27). By tackling housing quality head-on, policymakers bolster child health while stabilising communities—a win for both families and property markets.

6.8.4   Public-Private Partnerships for Nutrition

Improving child nutrition extends beyond distributing free school meals. Partnerships with supermarkets, local farms, and food distribution networks can reduce the cost of fresh produce in low-income neighbourhoods. Targeted subsidies for fruits, vegetables, and lean proteins—offset by levies on sugary foods—could replicate the success of public health initiatives observed in multiple high-income countries (28). Initiatives like universal breakfast clubs not only ensure children start the day nourished but also alleviate the morning stress on working parents, enhancing adult productivity and mental well-being.

6.8.5 Integrated Mental Health Services

Fragmented care frequently dooms children and teens to slip between the cracks of child and adolescent mental health services (CAMHS), primary care, and educational support. A more integrated system could tie school-based counsellors directly to community mental health teams, ensuring continuity of care even during transitions from primary to secondary school or beyond (29). Moreover, digital health innovations—like telepsychiatry and smartphone-based therapy modules—expand reach, especially in rural or underserved areas. However, bridging the digital divide remains crucial; technology can exacerbate inequities if not paired with free or subsidised broadband access.

6.8.6 Involving Local Communities

Policymakers can set the stage, but local communities must interpret and implement solutions in culturally and contextually relevant ways. Faith-based groups, youth-led organisations, and grassroots charities are often best positioned to identify children in distress early. Small grants and devolved decision-making can spur local innovations—community gardens, after-school tutoring, or mobile health vans—that address the specific barriers families face in a given locale. Research emphasises that community engagement fosters greater trust and higher uptake of public health measures (30).

6.9 Ensuring Generational Gains: Mechanisms of Accountability

6.9.1 Data-Driven Monitoring

One of the biggest pitfalls in child health policy is the lack of longitudinal, harmonised data to track progress. Creating an integrated child health index—covering everything from immunisation rates to housing stability, nutritional indicators, and educational milestones—provides real-time feedback loops for policymakers (31). If an area falls behind, targeted interventions can be deployed quickly. This transparency also helps voters hold politicians accountable, ensuring that pledges to tackle child inequities are monitored and validated by evidence rather than political spin.

6.9.2 Cross-Party Compacts

Given the long horizons needed for child health reforms to bear fruit, cross-party collaboration is pivotal. A Parliamentary Commission on Child

Health Inequality, for instance, could stipulate multi-year funding commitments insulated from election cycles. This approach aligns with successful models like the Swedish cross-party deals on education and healthcare, which have sustained consistent policy direction for decades (32). By removing child health from the short-term electoral tug-of-war, Britain secures stable, well-planned interventions that can weather political shifts.

6.9.3 Corporate Accountability and Social Investment

Private sector engagement can bolster or undermine child health efforts. From fast-food giants marketing to young audiences to property developers controlling rental prices, corporate activities shape the environment in which children grow. Encouraging corporate responsibility can include tax incentives for businesses that provide community health programmes, sponsor youth clubs, or adopt family-friendly work policies (33). Conversely, stiffer regulations might target industries that profit from unhealthy child-targeted products or exploit vulnerable families through predatory financial practices. Over time, responsible corporate behaviour can align market forces with social well-being, ensuring that child health is not trampled by profit motives.

6.10   Future-Proofing Britain's Social Fabric

6.10.1 The Moral Argument: Children Are Society's Common Responsibility

We often say, "It takes a village to raise a child." This adage underscores that child well-being is not a private affair but a communal one. A child who thrives contributes positivity to their community; a child who languishes out of neglect can inadvertently sow discord. The moral imperative is clear: no civilised society should tolerate gaping inequities in child health, especially when cost-effective interventions exist. If we fail at this fundamental moral level, the ramifications taint every subsequent societal relationship.

6.10.2 The Economic Argument: Invest Now or Pay More Later

The weight of empirical research suggests that a nation ignoring child health inequities is simply deferring, rather than avoiding, the economic burden (34). Conditions such as obesity, mental health disorders, and preventable chronic illnesses—rooted in childhood—metastasise into adult crises that cost billions in healthcare and lost productivity. Governments serious about long-term fiscal responsibility should see robust child health policy as not just a "social good" but a financial imperative. Early investment in children yields a compounding return, improving life trajectories and reducing welfare burdens.

6.10.3 Healing the Intergenerational Rifts

Addressing child health inequities can also function as a restorative act, rebuilding trust across generations. When older adults witness tangible improvements in youth services or family supports, they may feel reassured about their future care, seeing a more capable, stable younger generation stepping into economic roles. Meanwhile, younger families grappling with adversity sense they're not alone—that the system genuinely invests in their children's well-being. This virtuous cycle fosters renewed faith in institutions and fosters social solidarity.

6.11 A Different Tomorrow: Vision for an Inclusive, Vibrant Britain

6.11.1 Painting the Big Picture

Imagine a Britain where every infant can expect consistent healthcare screenings, nutritious meals, and stable housing. Schools become hubs of integrated services, offering tutoring, counselling, and extracurricular programmes that feed children's curiosities. Parents no longer choose between job security and adequate care for a sick child, because flexible work policies and community support structures lift that burden. Elders look upon the next generation with relief and optimism, confident that these young people, well-nurtured and well-educated, can sustain pension systems and innovate solutions to tomorrow's challenges.

This is not a utopian fantasy. Countries such as Finland, Denmark, and the Netherlands have demonstrated that strategic, early, and universal investments in children yield strong social cohesion, elevated academic performance, and robust economies (35). Britain's storied institutions—like the NHS—were once trailblazers. The question is whether Britain can once again reimagine its social contract, placing child well-being at its core.

6.11.2 Indicators of Success

Beyond raw GDP, Britain might measure success through child-centric indices: the proportion of children meeting developmental milestones, the decline in childhood obesity rates, or the fraction of adolescents who report a positive sense of mental well-being (36). Decreases in hospital admissions for preventable diseases or in the number of children living in temporary accommodation become national triumphs, not hidden footnotes. Over time, these metrics could steer policymaking, ensuring that child equity remains front and centre.

6.11.3   Global Implications

A fairer, more resilient Britain would serve as a beacon for other nations grappling with similar issues. If the UK can reverse rising childhood obesity, alleviate mental health crises among teens, and drastically reduce infant mortality in disadvantaged districts, it can once again export lessons on social policy innovation. Britain's potential role on the global stage—whether in negotiating trade deals or shaping developmental aid frameworks—gains credibility if it can demonstrate social harmony and robust health outcomes at home.

6.12   Conclusion: Rejecting the Myth of Separate Fates

Child health inequities form the invisible threads that tie together crises in adult mental health, elderly care, economic stagnation, and community unrest. Britain cannot treat these spheres as disconnected problems. Instead, they emanate from a single root cause: the systemic neglect of children's foundational needs. By allowing underprivileged children to flail, the nation undermines adults' financial stability, erodes older adults' security, and strains the very institutions meant to safeguard collective well-being.

Yet, a path forward is visible. With credible evidence at our disposal—ranging from PubMed-indexed analyses to large-scale cohort studies—policymakers, communities, and businesses can coordinate robust interventions. The cost of inaction is too high to ignore: creeping poverty, shrinking workforces, ballooning healthcare bills, and fractured social bonds. Conversely, the rewards of strategic investment are monumental. A generation nurtured with equitable healthcare, stable housing, mental support, and quality education will mature into adults capable of innovating, caring for elders, fuelling the economy, and reweaving the social fabric.

It falls to each citizen—whether a policymaker, educator, healthcare worker, parent, or concerned neighbour—to reject the myth that child health inequities exist in a silo. In truth, they are everyone's burden and everyone's crisis. Healing these rifts in childhood is not an act of charity; it is a commitment to forging a society in which prosperity, compassion, and sustainability echo through the life course. Only by making child well-being the shared axis of our policies, budgets, and cultural values can Britain truly shield itself from the grim future that awaits if we stand idle. We owe it to ourselves, our elders, and, most importantly, the generations yet to come to close the book on child health inequity—and write a new, inclusive chapter in Britain's history.

References

1. Marmot M, Allen J, Goldblatt P, Herd E, Morrison J. Build back fairer: the COVID-19 marmot review. London: Institute of Health Equity; 2020.
2. Heckman JJ. Skill formation and the economics of investing in disadvantaged children. Science. 2006;312(5782):1900–2.
3. Sen A. Development as freedom. Oxford: Oxford University Press; 1999.
4. World Health Organization. Constitution of the World Health Organization. Geneva: WHO; 1948. Basic Documents.
5. Bradley RH, Corwyn RF. Socioeconomic status and child development. Annu Rev Psychol. 2002;53:371–99.
6. Van Lancker W, Parolin Z. COVID-19, school closures, and child poverty: a social crisis in the making. Lancet Child Adolesc Health. 2020;4(5):e243–4.
7. Frith E. Children and young people's mental health: state of the nation. CentreForum; 2020.
8. Poulton R, Caspi A, Milne BJ, Thomson WM, Taylor A, Sears MR, et al. Association between children's experience of socioeconomic disadvantage and adult health: a life-course study. Lancet. 2002;360(9346):1640–5.
9. Felitti VJ, Anda RF, Nordenberg D, Williamson DF, Spitz AM, Edwards V, et al. Relationship of childhood abuse and household dysfunction to many of the leading causes of death in adults. Am J Prev Med. 1998;14(4):245–58.
10. Valle I, Gibb J, Gill C, Lucas P, Roberts H. Parental employment and child health and wellbeing. National Children's Bureau; 2013.
11. Patel V, Flisher AJ, Hetrick S, McGorry P. Mental health of young people: a global public-health challenge. Lancet. 2007;369(9569):1302–13.
12. Fuller AE, Shahidi FV, Comeau J, Wang L, Wahi G, Dunn JR, et al. Parental employment quality and the mental health and school performance of children and youth. J Epidemiol Community Health. 2025.
13. Lakasing E. Youth unemployment: A public health problem set to worsen if older people work longer. Br J Gen Pract. 2013 Jul;63(612):e506-7.
14. Gonäs L, Wikman A, Alexanderson K, Gustafsson K. Age, period, and cohort effects for future employment, sickness absence, and disability pension by occupational gender segregation: a population-based study of all employed people in a country (>3 million). Can J Public Health. 2019 May 14;110(5):584–94.
15. Lobstein T, Jackson-Leach R. Planning for the worst: estimates of obesity and comorbidities in school-age children in 2025. Pediatr Obes. 2016;11(5):321–5.
16. Institute for Fiscal Studies. The long-term costs of child poverty. London: IFS; 2016. IFS Commentary C125.
17. OECD. Education at a glance. Paris: OECD Publishing; 2021.
18. Wilkinson R, Pickett K. The spirit level: why greater equality makes societies stronger. London: Penguin; 2009.
19. Farrington DP, Welsh BC. Saving children from a life of crime: early risk factors and effective interventions. Oxford: Oxford University Press; 2007.

20. Nye JS Jr. Soft power: the means to success in world politics. New York: PublicAffairs; 2004.

21. Stiglitz JE, Sen A, Fitoussi JP. Mismeasuring our lives: why GDP doesn't add up. New York: The New Press; 2010.

22. O'Connell R, Knight A, Brannen J. Living hand to mouth: children and food in low-income families. Childhood. 2019;26(4):491–507.

23. Spencer N, Raman S, O'Hare B, Tamburlini G. Addressing inequities in child health and development: towards social justice. BMJ Paediatr Open. 2019 Aug;3(1):e000503.

24. Victora CG, de Onis M, Hallal PC, Blössner M, Shrimpton R. Worldwide timing of growth faltering: revisiting implications for interventions. Pediatrics. 2010;125(3):e473–80.

25. Weare K, Nind M. Mental health promotion and problem prevention in schools: what does the evidence say? Health Promot Int. 2011;26(suppl 1):i29–69.

26. Jacobs DE, Brown MJ, Baeder A, Sucosky MS, Margolis S, Hershovitz J, et al. A systematic review of housing interventions and health. J Public Health Manag Pract. 2010 Sep;16(5):S5–10.

27. Faresjo M, Faresjo T. The relationship between damp housing conditions and respiratory disorders in children: a cross-sectional study from the UK. BMC Public Health. 2020;20:1183.

28. World Health Organization. Fiscal policies for diet and prevention of non-communicable diseases: technical meeting report. Geneva: WHO; 2016.

29. Children's Commissioner. The state of children's mental health services. London: Office of the Children's Commissioner; 2020.

30. Haldane V, Chuah FLH, Srivastava A, Singh SR, Koh GCH, Seng CK, et al. Community participation in health services development, implementation, and evaluation: a systematic review of empowerment, health, community, and Process Outcomes. Maulsby C, editor. PLoS One. 2020;14(5).

31. Cowley S, Caan W, Dowling S, Weir H. What do health visitors do? A national survey of activities and service organisation. Public Health. 2007;121(11):869–79.

32. Bergqvist K, Yngwe MA, Lundberg O. Understanding the role of the welfare state in reducing inequalities in health. Int J Health Serv. 2013;43(3):415–32.

33. Kickbusch I, Gleicher D. Governance for health in the 21st century. Copenhagen: WHO Regional Office for Europe; 2012.

34. Doyle O, Harmon CP, Heckman JJ, Tremblay RE. Investing in early human development: timing and economic efficiency. Econ Hum Biol. 2009;7(1):1–6.

35. Bradshaw J, Richardson D. An index of child well-being in Europe. Child Indicators Res. 2009;2:319–51.

36. Children's Society. The good childhood report. London: The Children's Society; 2020.

7 Manifesto—The Hayre Doctrine

Introduction: A New Dawn in Child Health

Britain's children stand on an unsteady precipice. During times of crisis—from the global pandemic to austerity-induced budget squeezes—our youngest citizens are often the first to feel the tremors, yet the last to be considered in policy debates. For decades, patchwork measures have aimed to soften these injustices, but the same structural inequities keep resurfacing: skyrocketing child poverty rates, mental health crises among youth, housing insecurity, and uneven educational outcomes.

Following the seismic shocks of COVID-19, many have labelled the affected cohort as the "lost generation", referencing the enduring scars left by prolonged school closures, social isolation, and uneven digital access. A large body of empirical research, including systematic reviews indexed on PubMed, underscores the exacerbation of mental health disorders among children and adolescents during the pandemic (1,2). Economic analyses similarly reveal that disruptions in education and early-life care carry significant long-term costs, both for individuals and for society at large (3).

This manifesto—*The Hayre Doctrine*—advances a compelling new social contract, woven around a creative organising principle called *Hayre's Weighted Universalism*. In contrast to one-size-fits-all solutions, Weighted Universalism champions universal coverage of essential child services (healthcare, education, nutrition) with intensively scaled resources for children in situations of greatest adversity. By adopting this framework, Britain can transcend reactive, short-term policies and establish an equitable ecosystem in which every child has not just a theoretical right to thrive, but a real one.

Over the next sections, this manifesto will lay out the moral, economic, and social foundations of the Hayre Doctrine. We will see how integrating Weighted Universalism in everyday policy transforms child health from a patchwork of well-meaning efforts into a coherent, future-proof strategy. At its heart is a clarion call: A child's well-being is not a peripheral concern—it is the fulcrum upon which Britain's stability, prosperity, and moral standing rest.

DOI: 10.4324/9781003312529-8

7.1   Foundations of The Hayre Doctrine

7.1.1   The Moral Imperative

From the 1942 Beveridge Report to the creation of the NHS, Britain has a proud history of forging social policy in service of the vulnerable. Over time, however, moral imperatives have collided with austerity budgets, political short-termism, and uneven local implementation. The result is a stark reality: a rising generation of children left behind in substandard housing, lacking secure nutrition, or waiting interminably for mental health appointments (4). The pandemic further illuminated how these social determinants of health—especially poverty, education, and living conditions—can create enduring disparities in child outcomes (5).

The Hayre Doctrine reaffirms moral duty by enshrining *Hayre's Weighted Universalism* as the bedrock. This principle states:

> All children in Britain deserve universal coverage of core services, but those facing structural disadvantages—whether due to poverty, location, or additional needs—must receive proportionally greater assistance, ensuring that universal coverage does not become an empty slogan.

By guaranteeing universal access to healthcare, education, and nutritional support while layering extra resources in the communities that need it most, Weighted Universalism resolves the tension between "targeted" versus "universal" approaches. It becomes not merely a patch to fix problems but a moral statement: we cannot call ourselves a civilised society if we accept that a child's life chances should hinge on an accident of birth.

7.1.2   The Economic Imperative

Child health inequity is not only a breach of moral principle; it is also an unsustainable economic strategy. Research consistently shows that ignoring the basic developmental needs of children breeds heavy costs down the line: increased healthcare bills for chronic conditions, lost productivity when undernourished or uneducated children reach adulthood, and higher crime rates in communities plagued by hopelessness (6,7). The COVID-19 crisis further demonstrated the fragility of systems that deprioritise early-life investment: labour market shocks disproportionately affected lower-income families, and the resulting instability reverberated into children's mental health and educational outcomes (8).

Hayre's Weighted Universalism counters this wasteful cycle by front-loading investments—enabling early intervention in a child's life so that smaller, less costly solutions forestall far larger financial burdens. Governments operating under Weighted Universalism would see robust gains in workforce participation and tax revenue, while the reduced strain on social services frees up funds for other priorities. This synergy is both pragmatic and humane, distinguishing the approach from purely philanthropic or moral arguments. It integrates the well-known concept of "social returns on investment" but translates it into systematic, scaled policies aimed at dismantling structural barriers (9).

7.1.3 The Social Imperative

Societies torn by glaring child health inequities experience eroding trust and rising discontent (10). Working adults buckle under the care demands of children locked out of vital services, and the elderly worry who will fund pensions and staff care homes if younger generations are stunted. Community bonds weaken when resources shrink, and families feel forced to compete for scraps.

Weighted Universalism fosters cohesion by demonstrating that every child, in every neighbourhood, is precious enough to merit universal coverage, and every struggling family is worthy of deeper, targeted assistance. This dissolves the "us versus them" mentality that fosters resentment and cynicism. In turn, families are more likely to engage with local institutions—schools, clinics, youth centres—because they sense genuine respect for their experiences. By foregrounding equality of opportunity and emphasising structural solutions, the Hayre Doctrine sets a national tone of solidarity, reintroducing the ideal of a broad-based social contract in an era too often dominated by individualism and short-term political wins.

7.2 Redefining the Social Contract: The Pillars of the Doctrine

To operationalise the Hayre Doctrine, we propose five core pillars—*Universal Access, Early Intervention, Integrated Governance, Community Partnership, and Intergenerational Solidarity*—reimagined through the lens of Hayre's Weighted Universalism. These pillars trace a clear path for policymakers to design and implement innovative, evidence-based frameworks for child well-being.

7.2.1 Universal Access

Principle: All children in Britain must receive at least a universal baseline of healthcare, education, safe housing, and nutritional support. The Weighted Universalism twist is that baseline universal coverage includes additional "weights" for disadvantaged areas, ensuring equality of outcome rather than just equality of theoretical provision.

Healthcare: Establish free-at-point-of-use paediatric and mental health services—no more labyrinthine waitlists or geographic lottery. For children in high-poverty postcodes, Weighted Universalism channels extra GPs, nurse practitioners, and mental health counsellors, making universal coverage tangibly robust. Evidence from PubMed-indexed studies suggests that early, localised access to mental health care can significantly reduce adolescent depression and anxiety (11).

Housing: Guarantee stable, child-friendly accommodation as a non-negotiable right. Under Weighted Universalism, local councils receive scaled-up grants proportionate to the child homelessness rate, enabling proactive expansions in social housing. A longitudinal study demonstrated strong correlations between stable housing and improved child development markers (12).

Education: Extend universal early years places to all families, but intensify staff training and resources in schools serving large proportions of children on free school meals. "Universal" thus does not become "one size fits none", but a dynamic system that sends heavier aid where data indicates deeper deprivation. Evaluations of tiered educational approaches show that teacher–student ratios and resource intensiveness can dramatically affect literacy rates among disadvantaged cohorts (13).

7.2.2   Early Intervention

Principle: Swift, decisive action in a child's infancy or early school years can save families from the heartbreak of full-blown crises in adolescence.

Birth-to-Five Support: Weighted Universalism means universal home-visiting and robust nursery provision across the country, but with significantly more visits, staff, and programme expansions where data flags heightened vulnerability (e.g., teenage parents, low-income households, or care leaver families). Systematic reviews confirm that targeted home-visiting programmes consistently show positive outcomes in parent–child bonding, cognitive development, and maternal well-being (14).

Preventive Healthcare: Expand mandatory developmental screenings at frequent intervals—catching learning disabilities, speech delays, or early mental health problems. Weighted resources again go to areas with historically under-served populations. This approach aligns with existing calls from the Royal College of Paediatrics and Child Health to standardise child health checks nationwide (15).

Nutritional Safeguards: Introduce universal free school meals from nursery onward. In schools located in "nutritional deserts", Weighted Universalism mandates on-site dietician consultants and after-school cooking clubs to counter obesity or malnourishment. Research on school-based nutrition programmes indicates significant improvements in both BMI and educational performance when combined with parental engagement (1).

7.2.3 Integrated Governance

Principle: Siloed departments undermine synergy. Weighted Universalism emphasises cross-ministerial collaboration with an equity lens in budget allocations.

Child Equity Cabinet: A top-level governmental body merges decision-making from Education, Health, Housing, and Welfare, each adopting Weighted Universalism benchmarks. If a local authority has especially high child asthma rates, for instance, housing must prioritise mould eradication while healthcare officials intensify asthma clinics, and school boards roll out in-class air quality measures. This integrated approach resonates with the World Health Organization's call for "Health in All Policies" (16).

Single Assessment Portals: Parents fill out one integrated application for multiple benefits (housing, child benefit top-ups, mental health support) while Weighted Universalism calculates their "weight" of need. No more labyrinthine, repetitive form-filling, a process repeatedly criticised as a barrier to accessing services in high-income countries (17).

Legislative Filters: All new policies must pass a Weighted Universalism Impact Audit to confirm they do not reinforce child inequities. If negative impacts are detected, the policy is reworked or offset by proportionate compensatory measures. This Vancouver-style referencing approach ensures that child well-being remains a central criterion in legislative design, as recommended in wide-ranging child-health policy proposals (18).

7.2.4 Community Partnership

Principle: Local trust and grassroots creativity are indispensable in bridging the final mile between policy blueprint and child-level impact.

Neighbourhood Allies: Train local champions—mothers, faith leaders, retired teachers—who understand Weighted Universalism's resource scales and can guide families in tapping extra support. Similar community-based navigators have proven effective in maternal health programmes in Brazil and India, improving uptake of immunisations and antenatal care (19).

Participatory Budgeting: Weighted Universalism extends to local budgeting, letting communities vote on child-focused projects, with additional "weights" assigned where community metrics show higher child poverty or mental health concerns. Evidence from Porto Alegre, Brazil, highlights that participatory budgeting can lead to more equitable distribution of resources (2).

Cultural Partnerships: Engage cultural and religious institutions, distributing resources proportionate to the density of youth membership. They can host health fairs, tutoring sessions, or free meal programmes, all financed by Weighted Universalism grants reflecting local needs. Peer-reviewed papers on faith-based interventions in US communities demonstrate improved health literacy outcomes when cultural leaders take an active role (20).

7.2.5   *Intergenerational Solidarity*

Principle: The synergy between seniors, working adults, and children is essential. Weighted Universalism ensures each generation invests in the next, anticipating future returns that stabilise pensions, healthcare for older adults, and social tranquillity.

Elder-Child Co-Living: Weighted Universalism can reward housing initiatives where older adults share communal spaces with families, bridging the generational gap. Extra resources flow to projects that prove they reduce loneliness in seniors and enhance children's emotional security. A successful example is the intergenerational housing programme in the Netherlands, which shows mental health benefits for both parties (21).

Mentorship and Resource-Sharing: Pair older volunteers with families needing tutoring or child-care breaks; seniors earn small Weighted Universalism stipends if they provide consistent child-support hours in at-risk neighbourhoods. This model draws upon the concept of time-banking or service-exchange initiatives that have been piloted in some UK cities (22).

Long-Horizon Fiscal Benefits: Healthier children produce a more stable tax base in their working years, ensuring the next wave of caregivers and contributors for older generations. Weighted Universalism clarifies these direct links in all government communications—allowing seniors to see how supporting children secures the future of their own care.

7.3   Funding the Doctrine: Weighted Universalism in Action

One recurring question is how to pay for a universal approach that is also heavily scaled for at-risk populations. Weighted Universalism addresses this by establishing *flexible financing channels*—some innovative, some building on existing structures, yet all designed to funnel resources where they are most urgently required.

7.3.1   *Child Equity Fund*

National Pool: A dedicated Child Equity Fund aggregates revenue from progressive taxation (e.g., sugar taxes, minimal financial transaction levies) and philanthropic contributions. Weighted Universalism determines grant allocations: councils with high child poverty indices get proportionally larger funds. This mechanism mirrors the idea behind the "Fair Funding Formula", but with far more nuance (5).

Matching Mechanisms: Private corporations or local philanthropic groups can match public grants for specific Weighted Universalism programmes—like dietician expansions or after-school reading clubs. This synergy ensures local buy-in and sustained philanthropic interest, following successful precedents of blended financing in social welfare projects globally (23).

7.3.2 Social Impact Bonds and Partnerships

Social Impact Bonds (SIBs) can channel private capital into Weighted Universalism projects. If interventions reduce A&E visits or improve literacy rates in line with Weighted Universalism thresholds, investors receive modest returns from the savings accrued by local authorities. This harnesses market logic to social ends, ensuring that child-centred ventures can scale efficiently. While SIBs have been criticised for narrow outcome focus, Weighted Universalism mandates robust, multi-dimensional metrics that capture both short- and long-term benefits (24).

7.3.3 Universal Child Benefits with Weighted Tiers

Traditional universal child benefits remain essential, but Weighted Universalism refines them with targeted increments: families below certain income or housing thresholds receive a supplementary top-up, unlocking additional services. This approach is not "narrowly means-tested", because the universal baseline remains intact, yet it still ensures the greatest help goes to those who face the steepest obstacles (25).

7.4 Measuring Success: Data-Driven Accountability

Dedicating billions of pounds to Weighted Universalism without robust monitoring would merely perpetuate old inefficiencies. The Doctrine calls for a *sophisticated, transparent evaluation system* that can adapt policies based on real-world feedback.

7.4.1 The Child Equity Index

Multifaceted Indicators: BMI and vaccination coverage, yes—but also reading attainment, mental well-being surveys, stable housing metrics, and exposure to adverse childhood experiences. Weighted Universalism's success is gauged not by raw child counts served, but by progress bridging gaps between top-performing and worst-performing quintiles. The concept echoes the Marmot Review's emphasis on "proportionate universalism", but the Hayre Doctrine goes further (7).

Annual Child Parliament: A symbolic but powerful gathering where youth delegates from various localities present their lived experiences. They scrutinise official data and hold policymakers to account. Weighted

Universalism ensures delegates from deprived areas receive special travel stipends, guaranteeing diverse representation (26).

7.4.2   Parliamentary Reviews and Watchdogs

Child Equity Commission: Similar to the National Audit Office, but focused solely on child health and well-being. If Weighted Universalism allocations fail to reduce local obesity or truancy rates, the Commission can recommend mandatory improvements and resource re-allocation. Think of it as a permanent "Child Inequality Regulator" with real authority to force action.

Legislative Routines: Twice a year, ministers must deliver a Weighted Universalism Impact Update to Parliament. Constituencies see exactly how Weighted Universalism resources were deployed and what improvements or regressions emerged. This aligns with calls from child-rights advocacy groups for regular, transparent accountability measures (18).

7.4.3   Local Reflection and Recalibration

Community Scorecards: Weighted Universalism endorses community-level assessment. School councils or health boards release simplified "scorecards" rating local child health interventions, from playground safety to mental health wait times. This bottom-up accountability approach has been used effectively in some countries to measure local healthcare performance (3,27).

Adaptive Budgeting: If data show certain wards remain stuck in negative cycles—like high rates of childhood asthma—Weighted Universalism triggers an "intensive care" mechanism, directing a flood of extra resources and cross-agency interventions to that ward for a set period. Monitoring then tracks whether these concentrated injections of support raise child outcomes to match regional averages.

7.5   Cultural Shifts: Harnessing Creative Spirit

Policy frameworks alone cannot thrive if communities and individuals remain entrenched in outdated mindsets about child-rearing, resource allocation, and personal responsibility. The success of Weighted Universalism, therefore, hinges on cultural transformations parallel to structural reforms.

7.5.1   Destigmatising Poverty and Need

Weighted Universalism acknowledges that families in crisis aren't lazy or incompetent; they are battling social structures that hamper opportunity. By naming the phenomenon—'Hayre's Weighted Universalism'—and illustrating its rationale, we remove moral blame and recast it as a systemic solution.

Campaigns promoting this concept would highlight success stories: families who overcame adversity with the right help at the right time. Researchers of stigma in social assistance contexts have found that normalisation campaigns can reduce barriers to uptake (28).

7.5.2 Celebrating Children as Changemakers

Children aren't passive subjects of Weighted Universalism; they are co-creators. Schools can host "Idea Labs", letting children propose local solutions—like a weekend breakfast club or a pop-up community garden. Weighted Universalism funds the best ones proportionally, ensuring children in deprived areas see bigger budgets. This infuses a sense of agency, forging the next generation of civic-minded citizens. Studies on youth engagement in community health interventions show that children's input can dramatically increase programme relevance and uptake (29).

7.5.3 Bridging Social Divides

Widespread cynicism about "charity culture" or "handouts" can sabotage policy. Weighted Universalism defuses these tensions by clarifying that while services are universal, extra help goes where it's proven to be most needed—benefiting society as a whole. This distinction resonates with middle-class taxpayers and philanthropic donors alike, reaffirming that an equitable society invests more where the ground is rougher, not less. By integrating robust communication strategies, Weighted Universalism can foster empathy across class, geographic, and ethnic lines.

7.6 A Child's Journey Under Weighted Universalism

Consider Frida, a child born in a deprived coastal town. Traditionally, she might endure substandard housing, a stretched GP practice, and under-resourced schools. Under Weighted Universalism, her reality transforms:

1. **Early Health and Home Support:**
   Frida's parents receive routine home visits, universal to all families. Since her postcode ranks high on the Weighted Universalism deprivation index, they're offered additional parenting classes, rent assistance if eviction looms, and dietary advice from a local nutritionist. Randomised controlled trials support such enhanced visits in reducing child abuse and improving maternal life-course outcomes (14).
2. **Schooling with Scaled Benefits:**
   Entering primary school, Frida finds smaller class sizes, thanks to Weighted Universalism's staff expansions for high-poverty areas. Free school

meals include fresh produce from a local farmer's market, subsidised by Weighted Universalism grants. She also has a GP stationed part-time on site, ensuring quick checks for her chronic cough—mirroring a model seen in some Scandinavian contexts (30).

3. **Adolescence and Opportunity:**
   As a teenager, Frida benefits from robust extracurricular programmes— robotics clubs, sports, community-based mental health support—heavily funded for disadvantaged wards. Weighted Universalism ensures local employers receive tax credits if they hire or train local youth. Frida sees pathways beyond her immediate environment, fulfilling potential once stifled by poverty. Evaluations of vocational training schemes like Germany's dual education system underscore the capacity of bridging education and employment to break cycles of generational disadvantage (13).

This scenario exemplifies Weighted Universalism's life-course synergy, turning what once might have been a downward spiral into a ladder of opportunity.

7.7   Overcoming Obstacles: Navigating Resistance

7.7.1   Political Scepticism

Critics may label Weighted Universalism paternalistic, claiming it invests heavily in certain families. The Doctrine counters that standard universalism has historically done little to close the child health gap. Weighted Universalism aligns moral fairness with pragmatic resource distribution. By front-loading interventions where harm is greatest, it serves the long-term interests of everyone, including sceptics' own communities. Meta-analyses on early childhood education find returns frequently exceeding 7–10% per annum in social benefits (6).

7.7.2   Austerity Mindsets

A post-pandemic financial crunch might pressure the Government to revert to budget cuts. Weighted Universalism insists that scaling back on child equity is not "saving", but deferring staggering costs into the near future. Children robbed of decent nutrition or mental health support inevitably cost the NHS, schools, and welfare states multiple times over. Weighted Universalism's short-term resource intensification is dwarfed by the financial black hole created by adult crises that start in childhood.

7.7.3   Parental Autonomy Concerns

Some families may worry about state overreach. Weighted Universalism addresses these fears through an opt-in spirit: no family is coerced into interventions. However, universal baseline coverage remains non-negotiable, and additional support packages (like extra visits or community tutors) are offered rather than imposed. Parents retain autonomy, but Weighted Universalism ensures they cannot be left stranded by a hollow universal promise.

7.8 National and Global Dimensions

7.8.1 Reclaiming Britain's Moral High Ground

For decades, Britain's global brand rested on compassion-driven policies—NHS, universal education, robust social services. Child health inequities have tarnished that reputation. By adopting Weighted Universalism, Britain can restore itself as a template of progressive social policy. This moral leadership resonates in international forums—WHO, UNICEF, G7—positioning the UK as a champion of child-centred reform. Indeed, "Health for All" declarations, from the Alma-Ata to Astana, consistently stress that countries with equity-focused social policies not only improve outcomes but build resilience (31,32).

7.8.2 Enhancing Competitiveness

A generation of well-nurtured, mentally resilient children is the pipeline to a dynamic, knowledge-driven economy. Weighted Universalism invests early, ensuring each child enters adulthood with strong literacy, robust health, and flexible problem-solving skills. Globally competitive firms look for stable, skilled labour markets; Weighted Universalism can deliver precisely that, enticing new investments that see Britain as a cradle of top-tier human capital.

7.8.3 Exporting the Model

If Weighted Universalism thrives, it could spur a wave of policy emulation abroad—akin to the global ripple effect once prompted by the Beveridge Report. Countries wrestling with persistent child poverty might adopt or adapt Weighted Universalism as a proven formula for bridging inequality without sacrificing broad-based public support. This stands in contrast to other frameworks like "Universal Proportionalism" or "Conditional Cash Transfers" (7,27), which often fail to marry broad universal coverage with a systemic weighting that intensifies support precisely where it is needed most.

7.9 The Hayre Doctrine versus Existing Paradigms

To fully illuminate the novelty of the Hayre Doctrine, we must contrast it with established ideas—such as *Universal Proportionalism* (famously discussed in the Marmot Review) and unconditional universal programmes of the post-war welfare state.

1. **Universal Proportionalism (Marmot)**
   Marmot et al. emphasise proportionate universalism, where efforts are scaled by level of disadvantage (7). While the concept resonates with Weighted Universalism, the Hayre Doctrine explicitly codifies a more radical "heavy-lift" approach for those in the deepest poverty. It calls for not just "proportionate" scaling but also a *comprehensive re-evaluation* of funding channels, re-engineering them to saturate high-need areas with integrated interventions across housing, education, healthcare, and community development.

2. **Pure Universalism (Beveridge Tradition)**
   Traditional universalism (e.g., the universal healthcare premise of the NHS) is an invaluable baseline. However, stark inequalities in child health outcomes—especially since the 1980s—demonstrate that a single-tier universal model can inadvertently allow structural inequities to persist (10). Weighted Universalism's innovation lies in its formal system of "add-on weights", ensuring that areas of high deprivation receive proportionally **more** services, funding, and policy attention.

3. **Means-Tested or Targeted Interventions**
   Critics of universal approaches often push for exclusively targeted or means-tested benefits, citing cost-efficiency. Weighted Universalism transcends these approaches by combining the broad appeal and coverage of universal programmes with the ethical nuance of targeted scaling. The result is a "universal foundation" that leaves no child behind, but with additional tiers that thoroughly address entrenched disadvantage (25).

By distinguishing itself from these paradigms, the Hayre Doctrine cements its position as an *evolutionary leap* in social policy—a dynamic framework that blends moral clarity with data-driven, tiered resource allocation.

7.10   Conclusion: Seizing Our Defining Moment

Child health inequities are the canary in the coalmine—a stark warning that the very foundations of Britain's moral ethos and future workforce are at risk. *Hayre's Weighted Universalism* cements a radical yet deeply pragmatic ethos: not all children require the same intensity of help, but all deserve the baseline guarantee of thriving, and those on precarious ground deserve more.

   Within the ambit of the Hayre Doctrine, Weighted Universalism merges moral vision, economic prudence, and social inclusivity into one unstoppable force. The outcome is a triple win: children develop into confident, healthy adults; the workforce stabilises and innovates; and Britain's sense of community deepens. No longer do we accept illusions that a single-tier approach, or a purely means-tested approach, can solve child health inequities. Weighted Universalism ensures universal coverage is not just a policy fig leaf but a robust scaffold that lifts every child into a secure, dignified upbringing.

Now is the time to be bold. As the nation rebuilds after the pandemic, incremental measures won't suffice to close entrenched gaps. Weighted Universalism, anchored in this new social contract, offers a blueprint for a society that invests in its children not out of guilt or fleeting charity but out of a vibrant self-interest that unifies the moral, the economic, and the social into one luminous goal: a Britain where no child is left behind, no family is overlooked, and the entire population stands on the firm bedrock of inclusive opportunity.

Choose Weighted Universalism as our guiding star, and tomorrow's Britain emerges stronger, kinder, and more harmonious. Resist it, and we perpetuate a cycle of wasteful rescue missions and shattered prospects. The clarion call rings out: let us weave child health equity into the very fibre of our national identity, forging an era that future generations will recall as a turning point—the moment we declared that every child's promise was not negotiable.

This is the beating heart of the *Hayre Doctrine*—and it beckons all of us to answer its call with creativity, resourcefulness, and unwavering moral conviction. By ensuring that every child is equipped, protected, and empowered, we lay the cornerstone for a post-pandemic Britain that not only recovers but thrives, forging a legacy of justice, progress, and unity for generations to come.

References

1. Alaimo K, Olson CM, Frongillo EA. Food insufficiency and American school-aged children's cognitive, academic, and psychosocial development. Pediatrics. 2001;108(1):44–53.
2. Baiocchi G. Militant democracy: participatory governance in Porto Alegre, Brazil. Stanford University Press; 2005.
3. Björkman M, Svensson J. Power to the people: evidence from a randomized field experiment on community-based monitoring in Uganda. Q J Econ. 2009;124(2):735–69.
4. WHO Commission on Social Determinants of Health. Closing the gap in a generation: health equity through action on the social determinants of health. World Health Organization; 2008.
5. Implications of the National Funding Formula for schools. Education Policy Institute. 2017.
6. Heckman JJ. Skill formation and the economics of investing in disadvantaged children. Science. 2006;312(5782):1900–2.
7. Marmot M, Goldblatt P, Allen J, Boyce T, McNeish D, Grady M, et al. Fair society, healthy lives (The Marmot Review). The Marmot Review; 2010.

8. Pierce M, Hope H, Abel KM, Kontopantelis E, Webb RT, Ford T, et al. Mental health before and during the COVID-19 pandemic: a longitudinal probability sample survey of the UK population. Lancet Psychiatry. 2020;7(10):883–92.

9. Karoly LA, Kilburn MR, Cannon JS. Early childhood interventions: proven results, future promise. RAND Corporation; 2005.

10. Pickett K, Wilkinson R. The spirit level: why more equal societies almost always do better. Allen Lane; 2009.

11. Patel V, Flisher AJ, Hetrick S, McGorry P. Mental health of young people: a global public-health challenge. Lancet. 2007;369(9569):1302–13.

12. Hock ES, Blank L, Fairbrother H, Clowes M, Cuevas DC, Booth A, et al. Exploring the impact of housing insecurity on the health and wellbeing of children and young people in the United Kingdom: a qualitative systematic review. BMC Public Health. 2024 Sep 9;24(1).

13. Hanushek EA, Woessmann L. The knowledge capital of nations: education and the economics of growth. MIT Press; 2015.

14. Olds DL, Kitzman H, Cole R, Robinson J. Theoretical foundations of a randomized trial of home visitation by nurses. J Community Psychol. 2014;34(2):125–36.

15. Royal College of Paediatrics and Child Health. State of child health in the UK report. RCPCH; 2020.

16. World Health Organization. Health in all policies (HiAP) framework for country action. WHO; 2013.

17. Bradshaw J, Chzhen Y, Main G. The impact of the financial crisis on children. In: Farnsworth K, Irving Z, editors. Social policy in times of austerity. Policy Press; 2015.

18. Save the Children. Ensuring a healthy start for every child: policy proposals. Save the Children UK; 2020.

19. Victora CG, Barros FC, França GV, Da Silva IC, Carvajal-Velez L. The contribution of universal health coverage to sustainable development goals concerning maternal and child health in low- and middle-income countries. Int J Environ Res Public Health. 2022;19(5):2553.

20. Kaplan SA, Calman NS, Golub M, Ruddock C, Billings J. The role of faith-based institutions in addressing health disparities: a case study of an initiative in the Southwest Bronx. J Health Care Poor Underserved. 2006;17(suppl 2):9–19.

21. Verbeek-Oudijk D, van Campen C. Intergenerational cohabitation in the Netherlands: the association of changing demand and changing supply. J Hous Elder. 2017;31(3):295–308.

22. Seyfang G. Growing cohesive communities one favour at a time: social exclusion, active citizenship and time banks. Int J Urban Reg Res. 2003;27(3):699–706.

23. McKinsey & Company. The state of social impact investment. McKinsey Global Institute; 2017.

24. Fraser A, Tan S, Lagarde M, Mays N. Narratives of promise, narratives of caution: a review of the literature on social impact bonds. Soc Policy Adm. 2018;52(1):4–28.

25. Gregg P, Harkness S, Machin S. Child development and family income. Joseph Rowntree Foundation; 2009.
26. UNICEF. Child and youth participation resource guide. UNICEF; 2021.
27. Fiszbein A, Schady N. Conditional cash transfers: reducing present and future poverty. World Bank; 2009.
28. Baumberg B. The stigma of claiming benefits: a quantitative study. J Soc Policy. 2016;45(2):181–99.
29. Larson RW, Angus RM. Adolescents' development of skills for agency in youth programs: learning to think strategically. Child Dev. 2011;82(1):277–94.
30. Kodali PB. Achieving universal health coverage in low- and middle-income countries: challenges for policy post-pandemic and beyond. Risk Manag Healthc Policy. 2023 Apr 6;16:607–21.
31. World Health Organization. Declaration of Alma-Ata: international conference on primary health care. WHO; 1978.
32. World Health Organization. Declaration of Astana: global conference on primary health care. WHO; 2018.

Index